Collins

need to know?

Fertility & Conception

Professor Ian Greer

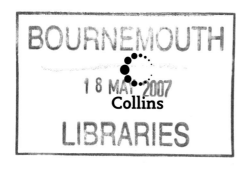

First published in 2007 by Collins
an imprint of
HarperCollins Publishers
77–85 Fulham Palace Road
London W6 8JB

www.collins.co.uk

Collins is a registered trademark of HarperCollins Publishers Ltd

09 08 07
3   2   1

A catalogue record for this book is available from the British Library

Editor: Emma Callery
Designer: Bob Vickers
Illustrator: Amanda Williams
Series design: Mark Thomson
Front cover photographs: © Alamy
Back cover photographs: © Getty Images

ISBN-10: 0-00-723622-0
ISBN-13: 978-0-00-723622-0

Colour reproduction, printed and bound by Printing Express, Hong Kong

Contents

1 Conception

It takes just one egg and one sperm to conceive, but getting them together is not always easy. Following sex, over 250 million sperm set off on a 'race' to find and fertilize the egg, but only one makes it all the way to the finish to enter the egg and trigger the whole process of making your baby. These are tough odds. But this is not the beginning, because producing the sperm and eggs is the culmination of complex processes in your and your partner's bodies, processes that must be carefully regulated by reproductive hormones (chemical messengers). So when starting to think about pregnancy perhaps the most logical starting point is to understand how your own body's reproductive system works.

The menstrual cycle

Regular menstrual bleeding is controlled by a complex system. The brain controls the release of 'signalling' hormones called gonadotrophins from the pituitary gland at the base of the brain. There are two gonadotrophins: follicle-stimulating hormone (FSH) and luteinising hormone (LH).

must know

Blood loss

Periods usually last for five to seven days. No matter whether periods are light or heavy, most of the blood is lost in the first three days. Average monthly blood loss is 30-40 ml (2-2¼ fl oz). Women with abnormally heavy periods lose over 80 ml (nearly 3 fl oz) of blood each time.

Ovulation

A woman is born with a lifetime's supply of eggs. During each menstrual cycle, FSH stimulates immature eggs contained in the ovaries to develop within small fluid-filled sacs known as follicles. Initially, several eggs begin to mature but generally only one continues to develop to full maturity. This is known as the 'dominant follicle'. Other eggs stop developing and disintegrate. When the egg is mature, the follicle it is contained within is about 2 cm (3/4 in) in diameter. As well as nurturing a developing egg, follicles also produce the female hormone oestrogen. When oestrogen levels are optimal and the egg is fully developed, the release of luteinising hormone (LH) occurs. This surge in the LH level triggers the release of the egg. This process is called ovulation.

Ovulation deals with egg production. However, if this egg is fertilized, it needs to implant in the womb. So it is important for the womb to be prepared for a fertilized egg, and oestrogen has a role here too. Oestrogen stimulates the lining of the womb (the endometrium) to grow and thicken. After the egg is released from the ovary, the remains of the follicle that released the egg produces a hormone called progesterone. (Progesterone is only made after an egg is released.) It acts on the lining of the womb by stopping its thickening at the right stage. It also improves the endometrium's blood supply and makes it a suitable and 'comfortable' environment for the fertilized egg to implant.

If a fertilized egg does not implant, the production of progesterone from the ovary falls sharply. As these hormone levels fall, the blood supply to the lining of the womb is reduced and the endometrium is shed. This results in the bleeding that we know as a period. The cycle then starts over again.

Time of ovulation

As ovulation (production of a mature egg) is essential for a regular menstrual cycle, women who have a regular cycle in the normal range (see right) are usually ovulating regularly. Conversely, women who do not ovulate regularly have irregular and usually infrequent periods.

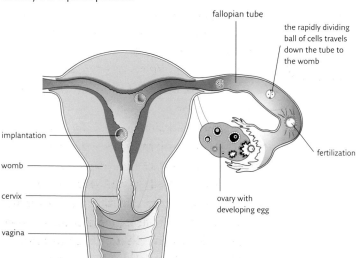

fallopian tube

the rapidly dividing ball of cells travels down the tube to the womb

Egg development through the menstrual cycle.

implantation

womb

cervix

vagina

ovary with developing egg

fertilization

The time of ovulation depends on the length of the menstrual cycle. If a woman has a 28-day cycle, ovulation occurs at around day 14, and if she has a 21-day cycle, ovulation occurs at around day 7 (see table, below). The time taken to mature an egg and ovulate can vary from woman to woman. The part of the cycle during which the egg develops is called the follicular phase, as the egg develops in a small 'follicle' or cyst in the ovary. However, the time from ovulation to a period (if fertilization does not occur) is fixed at around 14 days. This is called the secretary phase of the cycle as the ovary makes and 'secretes' progesterone. Provided your cycle is regular, you will be able to estimate when you will be ovulating.

Length of menstrual cycle (days)	Likely day when ovulation occurs
21	7
23	9
25	11
28	14
31	17
33	19
35	21

The optimum time of fertility

A woman is at her most fertile in the days around ovulation, and for a 28-day cycle this would be from days 12 to 15.

• To work out your fertile time, you need to estimate when ovulation will occur, which is usually 14 days before the first day on which your next period is due.

- For example, let's say that your period is due to start on 24 August. Take 14 days from 24 August and this is the date around which you will ovulate. In this example, it is 10 August.
- Once an egg is released, it remains viable for around a day. Allow a day or so on either side of this for minor variations in the time of ovulation. Sperm can remain viable in the woman's body for around two days.
- Therefore, the fertile time is estimated as being from two to three days before to two days after the estimated time of ovulation. This is the best time to try to conceive.

Some women know when they are ovulating because they feel lower abdominal pain at the time when the egg is released from the ovary. The pain is quite normal and is referred to as 'Mittelschmerz' (from German words for 'middle' and 'pain' – hence pain felt mid-cycle).

Typical timetable for a 28-day menstrual cycle

Day 1 Your period starts

Day 5 Your period stops

Days 1–14 The lining of the womb thickens under the control of oestrogen and the cervical mucous thins, making it easy for sperm to swim though

Day 14 Ovulation occurs

Days 15–28 As progesterone levels increase, the lining of the womb is prepared for a fertilized egg to implant

Day 26 Progesterone levels fall if implantation does not occur

Day 1 Your period starts

It's time to conceive

Many women wonder if they need to see their doctor for a health assessment before they conceive. However, no specific check-up is usually necessary if you are healthy, have no history of miscarriage, pregnancy complications or of a long-standing medical condition.

Stopping using contraception

If you have been using a form of contraception to prevent pregnancy, depending on what method this is, the length of time it might then take you to become pregnant is affected. Barrier methods do not disturb ovulation or the menstrual cycle and you can simply stop at any time. There is no need to delay attempts to conceive provided there are no other menstrual or medical problems.

If you use an intrauterine contraceptive device, or 'coil', for contraception then this must be removed before you try to conceive. It is probably best to delay conception until at least the next cycle as the coil may have disturbed the lining of the womb. So, after the doctor has removed the coil, you should use another technique, such as barrier contraception, until you are ready to conceive.

If you use the oral contraceptive pill or an injectable contraceptive, your normal menstrual cycle and ovulation is disrupted. The time from stopping the pill to ovulating is extremely variable. Estimates of the time of ovulation are based on the date when the next natural (not pill-induced) period is expected, so it is impossible to estimate when ovulation will occur after stopping the pill.

must know

Smear test
Check that your cervical smear tests are up to date before conceiving. If you need treatment for an abnormal smear, this should, ideally, be carried out before you get pregnant.

If you wish to get pregnant, it is best to stop taking the pill or injectable contraceptive and wait until your normal menstrual cycle resumes before trying to conceive. As this may take about three normal menstrual periods, you might want to use a technique such as barrier contraception until your cycle has stabilized. If you become pregnant before the regular rhythm of your periods has become established, this can make it difficult to predict your delivery date based on your last period. However, a reliable estimate of the stage of the pregnancy can be obtained with an ultrasound scan to measure the size of the developing baby (see pages 140–41).

Using your body temperature to predict ovulation

Your body temperature should fall slightly before ovulation then rise quickly afterwards. It is worth noting, however, that sometimes the fall prior to ovulation is absent. The increase in temperature occurs in response to the progesterone that is produced after ovulation occurs. Progesterone levels and the body temperature remain elevated until a day or so before the next period begins. If pregnancy occurs, the temperature rise (and elevated progesterone levels) persists.

• If you want to use this technique to find out when you are ovulating, take your temperature with a thermometer in the morning before getting out of bed. Any medical thermometer that can measure in tenths of 1 °C can be used. Thermometers (including electronic ones) and temperature charts can be purchased from pharmacies.

did you know?

Temperature change
• The typical change seen before ovulation would be a body temperature of 36.6–36.8 °C (97.9–98.2 °F), which falls to 36.2–36.4 °C (97.2–97.5 °F).
• The temperature would then increase to, say, 37–37.1 °C (98.6–98.8 °F) by around 36 hours after ovulation.
• If you regularly chart your temperature, you will see a pattern developing.

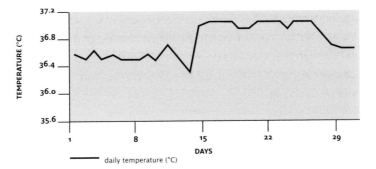

A typical pattern of temperature rise when ovulation occurs around day 14.

- If you are recording an oral temperature reading, remember to check your temperature before drinking anything hot or cold to avoid getting an inaccurate reading.
- Take your temperature at the same time every day.
- Repeat for each cycle that you want to check for ovulation. If you have a regular cycle, ovulation is likely to occur at around the same time during each cycle.

The downside of using this method to check for your fertile period is that your temperature rise occurs *after* ovulation and by the time your temperature has risen, the egg may no longer be viable. If you have a regular menstrual cycle, however, the time of ovulation may be anticipated based on a well-recorded pattern in temperature rise. This then allows intercourse to be timed to coincide with ovulation.

Consistency of vaginal mucous

The consistency of vaginal mucous can help predict the fertile phase as the character of the discharge varies through the menstrual cycle. Just after a period, it is scant, sticky and thick. Just before the time of ovulation, when oestrogen levels are high, the amount of mucous increases and it becomes watery, stringy and clear – a bit like raw egg white.

If you collect the mucous on your finger at this time and try to stretch it between your thumb and forefinger, it elongates for several inches without breaking. After the fertile phase, the mucous again becomes thicker. Sperm can survive particularly well in the thinner 'fertile' mucous, which also makes it easier for the sperm to get through the cervix and into the womb. So charting the pattern of changes in your vaginal mucous can also help you work out when you are ovulating.

Ovulation prediction kit

If you want to know when you are likely to be most fertile, you could buy an ovulation prediction kit. These kits, which are available from pharmacies, measure the amount of luteinising hormone (LH) – the hormone that stimulates the release of eggs from your ovaries each month – in your urine.

The kit identifies a surge in this hormone, which precedes ovulation by around twelve hours. This can help establish the fertile days in your cycle. Ovulation prediction kits are more accurate than temperature charts and avoid the need for regular temperature assessment, but they are also more expensive.

Frequency of intercourse

However, even with temperature charts or ovulation prediction kits, it is often difficult to identify the precise time of ovulation in advance. So, from a practical perspective, you should have intercourse several times around the estimated time of ovulation. Doctors have found that having intercourse once a week makes you 50 per cent less likely to conceive than having it every couple of days. Success rates do not appear to get significantly higher if you have sex every day. Sperm survives in the woman and is capable of fertilizing an egg for around two days after intercourse, especially during her most fertile time. In addition, there is no need to restrict intercourse at other times of the month. Indeed, the best plan is to have intercourse regularly every couple of days throughout the cycle. This avoids putting pressure on you both to identify the fertile time, obliging you to make love according to the calendar rather than by desire.

Sperm production

It is the same gonadotrophins that occur in women (follicle-stimulating hormone (FSH) and luteinising hormone (LH) – see page 8) that regulate sperm production in men. These hormones, or signalling molecules, are released from the man's pituitary gland at the base of the brain.

The sperm's journey

Follicle-stimulating hormone (FSH) stimulates the testicles to produce sperm – over 12 billion are produced each month. Luteinising hormone (LH) stimulates production of the male hormone testosterone within the testicles. Testosterone is essential for normal sperm production. After sperm are produced, they then have a long journey ahead before they are ready to fertilize an egg.

When they leave the testicles, they travel down a very fine coiled tube attached to the testicle called the epididymis, which is about 5–6 m (16–20 ft) long. Sperm entering the epididymis lack the ability to swim forwards, which is necessary to reach the egg. But as the epididymis sweeps them along, the sperm mature, so that by the time they reach the end of the epididymis, they have the ability to move or swim forwards. This whole process takes over 70 days.

Sperm are stored at the end of the epididymis. From there they flow into another tube, which connects the epididymis to the penis. This is called the vas deferens. This tube is about 30 cm (12 in) long and is coated in muscle. The sperm are propelled along the vas deferens by muscular contractions, and along the way they are mixed with seminal fluid produced from glands prior to ejaculation. This fluid is rich in nutrients to help keep the sperm alive and healthy after they are deposited in the vagina. This mixture of sperm and seminal fluid is called semen. About 2–4 ml (½–1 tsp) of semen containing many millions of sperm is released when ejaculation occurs. However, the sperm don't become completely mature until after ejaculation. It is only after ejaculation that they develop the capacity to break through the outer coating of the egg and fertilize it.

did you know?

Cool sperm
Sperm develop better at a temperature slightly cooler than the main body temperature, which is one reason why the testicles lie outside the body in the scrotum.

Male genital tract.

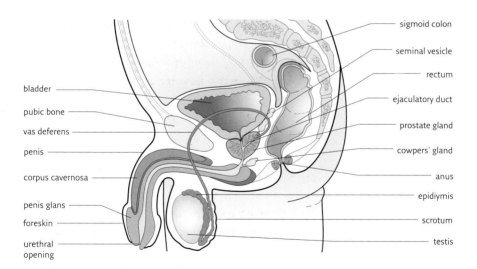

- sigmoid colon
- seminal vesicle
- rectum
- ejaculatory duct
- prostate gland
- cowpers' gland
- anus
- epidiymis
- scrotum
- testis

- bladder
- pubic bone
- vas deferens
- penis
- corpus cavernosa
- penis glans
- foreskin
- urethral opening

Conception

Normally a minimum of 40 million sperm are released with each ejaculation, but typically the quantity is over 80 million and often well in excess of 250 million. Although some are lost from the vagina, many make their way through the cervix (helped by the thin, watery mucous produced if the woman is fertile) into the womb and up into the fallopian tubes.

Egg meets sperm

The egg, having been released from the ovary, is picked up by the finger-like ends of a fallopian tube and transported down the tube. Fertilization of the egg occurs about one-third of the way down the fallopian tube. The egg is surrounded by sperm and eventually one sperm succeeds in penetrating the outer layer of the egg. This is the point of conception, after which no other sperm can penetrate the egg.

After conception, the genetic material (chromosomes) of the sperm and egg cells merge with each other and then the fertilized egg, which starts off as a single cell, divides to form two cells, then four, and then eight, and so on until a ball of cells is formed. This ball of cells continues its journey down the fallopian tube to the womb, where it stays for around three days, bathed in secretions from the womb.

About seven days after ovulation, it implants into the wall of the womb, whose lining has been prepared by the production of progesterone from the ovary (see pages 8–9). Another hormone, human chorionic gonadotrophin (hCG), is produced by the developing placenta. This maintains the production of progesterone from the ovary to help to support the early pregnancy.

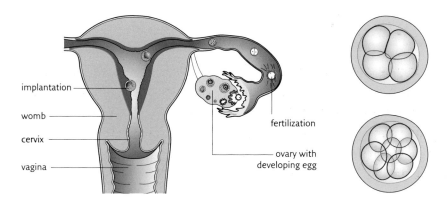

implantation

womb

cervix

vagina

fertilization

ovary with
developing egg

The ball of cells, once implanted, organizes itself into two different layers of cells, one that becomes the embryo and the other, the placenta.

Fertilized egg and cell division.

Genetic make-up and conception

All cells in the body contain DNA (deoxyribonucleic acid), the substance that makes up your genetic code. For this reason, DNA is sometimes referred to as the 'building blocks' of life. This is what makes you what you are, the blueprint for the structure and function of your body. Everyone except identical twins has a different genetic code. Your genetic code is made up of thousands of genes that are carried on 'chromosomes'. Each of us has 23 pairs of chromosomes in every cell in our body – a total of 46 chromosomes per cell. Of the 23 pairs of chromosomes in every cell, 22 pairs are 'general' chromosomes and one is a pair of 'sex' chromosomes.

Sperm and eggs are an exception to this general rule. An egg from a female has only 23 chromosomes; 22 of these are 'general' chromosomes and one is a 'sex' chromosome. The sperm from the male also has only 23 chromosomes: 22 general chromosomes and one sex chromosome. When conception occurs and the sperm

1 Conception

fertilizes the egg, the egg and sperm cells fuse. A fertilized egg therefore has the full complement of 46 chromosomes and the baby that grows from the egg has 46 chromosomes in every cell.

The sex of the baby conceived is determined by the 'sex' chromosomes – referred to as 'X' and 'Y' chromosomes – and the way these combine determines whether we are male or female. All girls have two X chromosomes and no Y chromosome, while a boy has one X and one Y chromosome. It is the sex chromosome that comes from the father's sperm that determines the sex of your baby. The mother has no power to influence the sex of the baby because she can contribute only an X chromosome, whereas the father can contribute either an X or a Y chromosome.

**A normal karyotype: The chromosomes, which carry the genetic code are laid out in their pairs.
Down's Syndrome: The karyotype of a person with Down's Syndrome has an extra chromosome 21–3 instead of 2.**

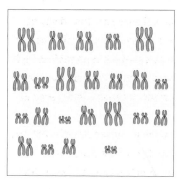

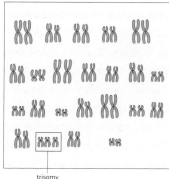

trisomy

standard human karyotype

down syndrome karyotype

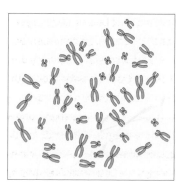

random arrangement of karyotypes in cell

Sexual position and conception

Provided intercourse is comfortable and semen is deposited at the top of the vagina, the sexual position should not influence conception. However, it is perhaps best for the woman to avoid more upright positions after the man ejaculates to prevent some of the semen draining out of the vagina, although there is no evidence that resting after intercourse increases the likelihood of pregnancy. Equally, there is no truth in the old wives' tale that you can't get pregnant if you have intercourse standing up.

Age and conception

There is no 'ideal' time to get pregnant. Fertility varies from person to person, although fertility in both men and women reaches its peak at about the age of 24 years. Many women are now delaying pregnancy until their 30s and even 40s where, once over the age of 35, they are at greater risk of developing complications such as high blood pressure during pregnancy. If you are over 35 years old, there is also a higher risk of chromosomal problems in the fetus, such as Down's syndrome.

It is not just older mothers who are at increased risk of problems. The risk of complications is also higher if you have a pregnancy when you are a teenager. So, from the doctor's perspective, having your babies somewhere between the age of 20 and 35 is best in order to minimize the risk of complications, some of which can be serious. However, you may not be at a stage in your life when you can have your babies at that time. So do remember that the majority of women over 35 have a successful pregnancy outcome. It is important to keep these extra risks associated with age in perspective, but seek medical advice if you have any particular concerns and, in particular, if you have an existing medical problem. The 'best' time to become pregnant depends largely on what is best for you and your partner, taking into account and weighing up everything that is going on in both your lives and thinking about what pregnancy will mean for you.

2 A healthy pregnancy

Every woman knows that it is really important to take good care of her health when she is pregnant. But many women are not aware that their health before pregnancy is critical to producing a healthy baby. This means that you need to think about your health and, in particular your diet, not just after that positive pregnancy test, but for several months before.

Your pre-pregnancy health

Doctors have known for a long time that pre-pregnancy care is important. Although women are becoming increasingly health conscious and some now seek specific pre-pregnancy advice, there are many women who don't understand its importance.

Take care of yourself

We all lead hectic lives and all too often missing your first period is the catalyst for thinking about your pregnancy, but you are already two weeks pregnant at this point and it may take a further few weeks before you see your obstetrician. By this time, your baby is developing rapidly and you may have missed opportunities to influence the pregnancy positively.

• The first twelve weeks of pregnancy is the time when all of the major organs are developing in the baby's body.

• The heart, lungs, liver, kidneys, brain and nervous system are all formed at a time when many women do not even realize that they are pregnant.

This is why pre-pregnancy care is so important. It is important not just for women with a health condition, but for every woman contemplating pregnancy.

Your diet

If you are thinking about becoming pregnant, diet is important. It has been said that you are what you eat and, of course, your baby will be too. Indeed, eating a well-balanced diet before you conceive is one of the most important things you can do for your baby. For more information, see pages 26-47.

Your weight

In addition, if you are overweight, it is best to reduce your weight before trying to conceive. This is because not only does being overweight reduce your chances of conceiving, but it also puts you and your baby at greater risk of many complications. For more information, see pages 52–3.

Smoking

If you are a smoker, you should know that smoking can not only reduce your fertility, but also make you more prone to miscarriage and restrict your baby's growth in the womb. Stopping smoking is easier said than done and it may take you some time to give up smoking completely. Ideally, you and your partner should try to stop several months before attempting to conceive. You should also know that it is never too late to stop. Stopping smoking even after you are pregnant can make a difference for your baby. For more information, see pages 44–5.

Be aware of your surroundings

If you work with certain chemicals, lead, anaesthetics or X-rays, this may involve a risk to your unborn baby. Talk to your doctor about it. It has been suggested that computers, visual display units (VDUs) and copying machines give off harmful rays encouraging miscarriage, but despite several large studies there is no scientific evidence to suggest that they present any risk to pregnant women or their babies. Other studies on women who delivered small babies have likewise identified no link between VDU exposure and low birth weight. So if you work with a VDU, there is no need to be concerned or to take any special precautions when you are pregnant.

did you know?
Conception and stress
If you have been trying desperately for a baby and you have not conceived, you can end up feeling stressed and anxious, which can have an adverse effect on conception. Having a balanced diet, getting enough sleep and taking regular exercise should help. If you have a very stressful occupation, you might want to consider ways of limiting or avoiding stress at work.

Your diet

Diet is fundamental to good health, and no more so than when you are preparing for pregnancy or in early pregnancy. All the 'building blocks' of your baby's body are derived from your food.

A balanced diet

A balanced diet provides you with:

- protein for muscles and other structures
- calcium for bones
- carbohydrates for energy
- fats for cell growth
- vitamins for key body functions

An optimal nutritional balance is the first step to giving your baby the best start in life. The requirements for protein, iron, calcium and vitamins B, C, D and E increase in pregnancy, but a well-balanced diet usually provides you with enough protein, vitamins and minerals to meet these extra demands.

Your baby's health depends to a great extent on the health of not only you but also your partner at the moment of conception. You increase your chances of conceiving a healthy baby if you both eat a healthy, varied diet. Ideally, you should keep your intake of foods rich in fat and sugar to a minimum and your diet should include:

- a good selection of fresh vegetables and raw fruit (taking care to wash them thoroughly) to provide vitamins and fibre
- foods rich in protein, such as lean meat, fish, poultry, eggs and beans
- foods rich in calcium, such as milk, cheese and yoghurt

must know

Meal times

Eat regular meals with a wide variety of healthy foods that you enjoy. If you get your diet right before conception, you will have established an ideal pattern for your pregnancy.

• cereals, bread, pasta and potatoes to provide carbohydrates and additional fibre

It is also sensible to combine this diet with an adequate fluid intake. Water is better than coffee, tea or sugar-rich drinks, such as cola.

Fruit and vegetables

Try eating more salads using a wide range of fresh vegetables, and try to take two portions of vegetables or fruit with each meal. Avoid over-cooking vegetables as this breaks down many of the vitamins they contain; try steaming them instead. Have fresh (not canned) fruit for dessert and drink fruit juices.

Protein

You can get most of your protein from meat like chicken, beef and lamb as well as nuts and pulses, but fish is an excellent source of protein, and oily fish like salmon and herring are rich in essential fatty acids (so-called omega 3 essential fatty acids), which are important for the development of the baby's brain and nervous system. Moreover, a high fish intake is associated with a reduced risk of pregnancy complications such as premature labour or a low-birth weight baby. That said, there are some fish that should be avoided if you are trying to conceive or if you are pregnant (see page 37).

Calcium

Foods rich in calcium such as milk, cheese and yoghurt are important to eat to ensure you have good calcium stores for the developing baby. When you are pregnant, drinking 500 ml (18 fl oz) of milk per day or 250 ml (9 fl oz) of milk and eating a yoghurt or portion of cheese is enough to ensure that you have sufficient amounts of calcium in your diet.

Carbohydrates

These are essential for energy. Many women worry about carbohydrates being related to weight gain and thus cut down on all forms of carbohydrate when trying to become pregnant. There are 'good' and 'bad' types of carbohydrate, however. Starchy foods such as pasta, wholemeal bread and potatoes are 'good'. 'Bad' carbohydrates are sugar-laden foods, such as cakes, biscuits and sweets. Cut down on these and think about increasing your intake of starchy carbohydrates. You should try to eat wholemeal bread, and take a portion of potatoes, pasta or wholegrain rice with each main meal. For breakfast think about having porridge or a high-fibre or wholegrain breakfast cereal, and avoiding cereals with a high sugar content.

Fibre

Otherwise known as 'roughage', fibre is found in foods derived from plants. It cannot be easily digested and absorbed by our bodies and so it stays in the bowel, providing roughage. It can be broken down to some extent by bacteria in the large bowel and some of these breakdown products can be absorbed and used as a source of energy. Because it provides roughage for the bowel – aiding the process of peristalsis (contractions in the bowel) by which the food is pushed through the gut. Fibre is important in ensuring that bowel function is normal and in preventing constipation. This is especially important in pregnancy when your bowel function often slows down. Many women thus find constipation a problem during pregnancy, and eating a fibre-rich diet is very good at preventing this.

You should therefore eat foods with a high-fibre content, such as wholemeal bread, pasta and fruit. However, if you increase your fibre intake suddenly, you may find that you feel bloated and have excess wind, so it is better to increase your intake gradually. You should also 'match' the increase in fibre with an increase in fluid intake, preferably water.

Fluid

It is all too easy to get slightly dehydrated. We have busy lives and often drink too much caffeine in tea and coffee that can add to the dehydration. It is a good idea to increase your fluid intake. You should aim to drink around six glasses of water a day. In pregnancy you will be prone to constipation as the bowel tends to become more sluggish because of the effect of pregnancy hormones, so along with an increase in fibre in your diet, drinking water helps to prevent constipation.

Reducing fat intake

It is best to avoid fried food and foods with a high fat content such as meat pies, sausages and pastries. If you want to fry food, then cook it in unsaturated vegetable oil, such as olive oil, or try grilling it instead. You should choose lean meat and trim off any excess fat before you cook it.

Reducing sugar intake

When pregnant, you should avoid high levels of sugar in your diet. Try to avoid or at least minimize your consumption of sweets and chocolate and also sugar-rich soft drinks. It is, of course, easier said than done, but try to eat fruit for a snack instead, and drink mineral water.

Reducing salt intake

You do not want or need to eliminate all salt from your diet. Moderation is the key: try not to put extra salt on the foods you eat and minimize the salt you add during cooking, as well as eating fresh foods rather than processed or tinned products, which are often high in salt. Meat extracts and soy sauce are high in salt, too, so keep intake of these to a minimum.

Vitamins and minerals

A regular intake of vitamins C and D are important both before and during pregnancy. In a well-balanced diet, it should be possible to obtain the necessary quantities without resorting to vitamin supplements. In fact, the only vitamin supplement that is usually needed before and during pregnancy is folic acid (see pages 33–6). Specific supplements of vitamins C and D are not usually required prior to pregnancy unless you have particular medical or nutritional problems, in which case you need to seek advice from your doctor. If you are vegetarian or vegan, you may need specific supplements of vitamins and minerals. These, too, require individual advice from your doctor.

Vitamin C

Available from fresh fruit and vegetables, vitamin C is important as it helps you absorb iron and also because it is needed for the production of the red blood cells that carry oxygen around the body. In pregnancy, there is a significant increase in the number of red blood cells in a woman's body – around 25 per cent on average by 32 weeks of pregnancy. So there is an extra demand for vitamin C, iron and folic acid, not just for the baby but also for the mother as all these vitamins and minerals are essential for red blood cell production.

Vitamin D

Vitamin D is essential for the good development of bones. It is available from dairy products.

Vitamin A

Too much of certain dietary component can sometimes cause potential harm. When it comes to vitamins in pregnancy, vitamin A is one to know about. Vitamin A is a fat-soluble vitamin that is stored in your liver and it is vital for the maintenance of good eyesight, and healthy skin, hair and nails. In the developing baby, vitamin A is essential for tissue growth.

Vitamin A occurs in two main forms in our diet: the first form is 'retinol' – the 'real' vitamin A; the second is the 'carotenoids', which your body converts into retinol. Beta-carotene is a carotenoid and is converted into retinol only when it is required. It acts as an antioxidant in the body (helping to prevent damage to blood vessels caused by free radical molecules) and is the pigment that gives the green, yellow or orange colour to vegetables and fruit. The brighter the vegetable, in fact, the more beta-carotene it contains. Fresh liver is a particularly rich natural source of vitamin A, as animals, like humans, store vitamin A in their livers.

Very high intakes of 'true' vitamin A – 'retinol' – have been linked with an increased risk of fetal abnormalities during pregnancy. Such high levels are likely to be far in excess of those you would find in your normal diet, however. The amount of retinol linked with fetal abnormalities is in excess of 3,300 mcg per day. This level is very high: you would need to eat 30 eggs in one day, for example, to get that much vitamin A. At the same time, you should not take supplements containing vitamin A in the retinol form or eat foods that are very rich in retinol, such as liver or liver products like pâté, when you are planning to become pregnant or are pregnant. Similarly, fish liver oils (e.g. cod liver oil) should also be avoided.

must know

Foods containing vitamin A
- liver
- liver pâté
- carrot
- full fat milk
- egg

must know

Women who are likely to have low iron stores
• vegans /vegetarians
• those who have had two or more pregnancies close together
• those who have suffered from anaemia
• those with heavy periods
• those who are expecting twins, triplets or more

must know

Foods containing iron
• breakfast cereal
• red meat
• baked beans
• green leafy vegetables
• eggs
• wholemeal bread

Iron

Iron is a mineral that is stored in your liver, spleen and in the centre of certain bones. Maintaining an adequate iron intake is important both before and during your pregnancy. Your developing baby needs iron for the formation of several important proteins. In particular, iron is required for the formation in the red blood cells of haemoglobin, the substance that transports oxygen around your body.

If you have an adequate intake of iron in your diet before and during your pregnancy, you are usually able to meet your own and your developing baby's needs. Iron supplements are not routinely required when planning a pregnancy. However, there are some women who are more likely to have low iron stores and therefore need to take supplements. These include women who had low iron stores or a diet poor in iron before pregnancy and women expecting twins or triplets (see also page 141). Your doctor is able to advise you about this.

You find iron in foods such as baked beans, bread (fortified white, as well as brown and wholemeal), breakfast cereals, pulses (such as lentils and red kidney beans) and red meat (but avoid liver because of its high vitamin A content).

If you require iron supplements, you can maximize the absorption of iron by taking the iron tablet with a citrus drink such as fresh orange juice, which is rich in vitamin C (also important for treating anaemia).

If you suffer from heartburn or indigestion, do not take the iron supplements at the same time as antacid medicine as this reduces the absorption of iron. In pregnancy, iron supplements are often combined with folic acid, frequently in the same tablet.

Folic acid

Folic acid is an important member of the B vitamin family and, as such, is essential in small quantities for maintaining normal body metabolism. Because folic acid does not occur naturally in your body you need to obtain it from other sources such as your food or by means of vitamin supplements.

The importance of folic acid

Folic acid is essential for the production of healthy red blood cells, which carry oxygen around the body. We are constantly making and replacing our red blood cells: it has been estimated that, on average, an adult makes more than 120 million new red blood cells every minute throughout their lives. Hence deficiency of folic acid means that an insufficient number of red blood cells are produced, leading to problems such as anaemia.

Folic acid is also known to reduce the risk of certain abnormalities in the baby known as neural tube defects, of which spina bifida (which in its severe form can be seriously dangerous for the baby), is perhaps the best known. All babies are potentially at risk of spina bifida, or other neural tube defects such as hydrocephalus, whatever the mother's age and whether or not this is a first or a subsequent pregnancy.

The neural tube is the part of the developing baby that eventually becomes the brain and the spinal cord. It forms at about four weeks after conception or about two weeks from the time of a missed period. Research has shown that sufficient folic acid in the mother's blood is essential for normal formation of the neural tube. Interestingly, in the USA, folic acid has been added to all flour for bread and pasta from 1998. Since that time, the number of babies with neural tube defects has fallen by

watch out!

There is one relatively uncommon form of anaemia due to deficiency of vitamin B12. Folic acid supplements could make it difficult for routine blood tests to pick up this condition. If you have a history of anaemia due to vitamin B12 deficiency, check with your doctor before taking folic acid.

almost 20 per cent. There is also some evidence that suggests that adequate folic acid intake might help prevent problems such as small-for-dates babies.

Spina bifida and hydrocephalus

In babies with spina bifida there is a defect in which part of one or more vertebrae (the bones making up the spine) fails to develop completely, leaving a portion of the nervous tissue in the spinal cord exposed, which leads to damage of the nerves. This defect can occur anywhere in the baby's spine but is most commonly seen in the lower back. The condition varies in severity and much depends on where the defect is and how much of the nervous tissue is exposed. Mild cases may have no major disability but in more severe cases, there can be paralysis of the legs, loss of sensation and incontinence due to loss of bladder control.

Women who have had a child with spina bifida are more at risk than women who have had a child without the condition. In such instances, it would be worthwhile obtaining specific pre-pregnancy advice before conceiving again, and you should consult your doctor.

Hydrocephalus is where there is an excess of fluid in chambers within the brain. This often arises because the flow of fluid through these chambers is obstructed. The excess fluid builds up in the chambers and the pressure causes them to enlarge, which can damage the brain tissue. Hydrocephalus may occur with spina bifida or on its own.

Folic acid from supplements

The ideal time to start taking folic acid supplements is two to three months before starting trying to conceive. Make it a part of pre-pregnancy planning. The tablets can be obtained from all good pharmacies. If you don't like taking tablets, try folic acid milk, also available from pharmacies; one carton usually represents the daily requirement. Always remember to follow the instructions on the pack carefully. If you are taking prescribed medicines, check with your doctor before taking any supplements to be on the safe side.

Folic acid from food

Folic acid is soluble in water and is stored mainly in the liver. It is largely destroyed by cooking, however, so serve salads and stir-fry or steam vegetables lightly rather than boiling them. You can obtain it from:
• fresh dark green vegetables like broccoli, Brussels sprouts, peas, green beans, chick peas and spinach
• oranges
• peanuts, although salted peanuts should be avoided if possible because of the extra salt. In addition, if you or your family has a history of peanut allergy or other allergic conditions, like asthma and hay fever, it is definitely recommended that you avoid peanuts during pregnancy
• many breakfast cereals have added folic acid (read the label) and milk and yoghurt also contain it
• wholemeal and wholegrain breads are high in folic acid, as are wheatgerm, brewer's yeast and yeast extract, so add these to your diet

Many women with a healthy diet may already have a sufficient folic acid intake for pregnancy simply from their food without the need for supplementation. But folic acid deficiency commonly arises in pregnancy due to the many extra demands the development of the baby places on the mother's body. Even women who have an adequate diet may not be taking in sufficient amounts of

must know

Folic acid allowance
• The recommended daily allowance for adults is 200mcg, but prior to becoming pregnant it is recommended that the intake is doubled to 400mcg a day.
• Continue to take 400mcg for at least the first 12 weeks of your pregnancy.
• Some doctors are happy for you to stop while others recommend you take it throughout pregnancy – folic acid is a vitamin that can help prevent health problems such as anaemia and might help to reduce any other pregnancy complications.

folic acid because the body is not absorbing it efficiently from food.

Folic acid supplements are therefore recommended for every woman trying to conceive to be sure that her intake is sufficient. In pregnancy, the kidneys filter folic acid from the blood at four times the normal rate, which is another reason why supplements are recommended. If you decide not to take folic acid supplements, however, ensure that you have a good daily intake of folic acid in your diet by eating suitable quantities of the foods listed on the previous page.

Foods to avoid

There are certain foods that are best avoided when you are trying to conceive and also in pregnancy. This is because of the risk of infection or because they contain potential toxins.

For example: unpasteurized milk, soft cheeses and pâté can contain a type of bacteria called listeria that can cause miscarriage and premature labour; raw and uncooked cured meats (such as ham and prosciutto) and unwashed (soil-covered) vegetables may carry toxoplasma, an organism that can cause abnormalities in the baby (see pages 46–7). Liver contains high quantities of vitamin A (see pages 30–31); and raw meat, poultry and eggs can carry salmonella, a type of bacteria that causes food poisoning.

Processed food

It is all too easy to rely on processed food from time to time when we have busy lives. But try if possible to avoid convenience foods that have been highly

watch out!

When storing or preparing food, remember to keep raw meat and poultry separate from cooked or pre-prepared foods and use separate utensils for them. In addition, always wash your hands thoroughly after handling raw meat and poultry.

processed, such as canned foods and packet mixes. This is because these often have added sugar and salt as well as a high fat content. So if you have been taking care of what you eat and limiting salt and sugar intake, you might be unwittingly undoing the benefits of your efforts by eating processed pre-prepared food. These foods may also contain chemicals in the form of artificial flavourings, colourings and preservatives. The composition and additives in these foods can usually be identified by looking at the label.

Fish

A US food and drug administration panel has recently recommended that pregnant women should limit their consumption of those fish that are at the top of the food chain. So you should not eat a lot of tuna, and completely avoid swordfish, shark, tilefish and king mackerel. This is because of concerns that these particular fish may contain levels of mercury that could be harmful to people, especially developing babies.

Mercury enters the sea environment through pollution and virtually all fish contain tiny amounts of mercury. Long-lived fish that are predators, such as sharks or swordfish, accumulate the greatest amounts of mercury in their bodies and so might be harmful to people who eat them regularly. The safe level of tuna intake with regard to the effects of mercury in pregnancy has not been established, but in the meantime it has been recommended that pregnant women should eat no more than two 175 g (6 oz) cans of tuna each week, just to be on the safe side.

must know

Foods to avoid eating in pregnancy
- unpasteurized milk and milk products such as soft and mould-ripened cheeses
- pâté
- raw and uncooked cured meat
- unwashed fruit, vegetables and salads
- raw or partially cooked eggs
- raw shellfish
- liver
- liver sausage
- dietary supplements rich in vitamin A, e.g. cod liver oil
- shark, swordfish, king mackerel

Vegetarian and vegan diets

More and more people are turning to vegetarian or vegan diets. Some vegetarians eat dairy products and others eat dairy products but avoid eggs. Vegans avoid all animal products including meat, fish, dairy products, eggs and honey. Because a few micro-nutrients occur naturally only in animal products, planning a balanced vegetarian or vegan diet requires a little extra effort. There are not usually any problems with a well-balanced vegetarian diet before and during pregnancy, however. Such a diet provides sufficient protein, vitamins and minerals to meet the needs of most women, although sometimes iron supplements are required to help prevent anaemia caused by the extra demands of the unborn baby on the mother's stores of iron.

Some very strict vegan diets contain no food at all that is derived from animal sources, including dairy products. Women following such a diet may need extra vitamin supplements and should discuss this with their GP. If you are a vegan, you may be prescribed supplements of calcium and vitamins D and B12. So there are not usually any problems with a well-balanced vegetarian diet during pregnancy; indeed, you will have some benefits, such as increased fibre in your diet from all the fruit and vegetables.

The quantity of food

How much food you need to eat depends on your body weight and BMI (see page 49) and also on how much exercise you take (see pages 56–63). However, if your BMI is in the healthy range for your age, typical servings per day of popular foods are as follows:

- one to two 75–110 g (3–4 oz) servings of lean meat
- six portions of fruit and vegetables, such as a medium-sized apple or peach or three heaped tablespoons of a vegetable
- five slices of wholemeal bread
- one to one and a half portions of rice (75 g (30 z)) or pasta (110 g (4 oz))
- one serving (medium bowl) of unsweetened breakfast cereal
- 600 ml (1 pint) of milk or a 300 ml (½ pint) of milk and a yoghurt or serving (around 25 g (1 oz)) of cheese is enough to meet a pregnant woman's extra calcium needs

In addition, a portion (150 g (5 oz)) of fish can be eaten every other day

In late pregnancy, however, increase your energy intake by about 10 per cent, which amounts to an additional 200 calories for the average woman. This amount of calories can be gained by eating a large bowl of cornflakes with semi-skimmed milk, or two medium slices of wholemeal bread, very lightly buttered, although the amount can be spread out over several smaller meals if a large portion cannot be eaten in one sitting at this stage of pregnancy.

Dieting

Going on a diet to lose a lot of weight is not advisable or recommended immediately before or during pregnancy. This is because you may disturb your nutritional balance at crucial stages of your baby's development. However, limiting weight gain in pregnancy is important for women who are overweight and this can be achieved by carbohydrate restriction, ensuring that you take no more than the recommended number of servings of carbohydrate in your daily diet. (See also page 28.)

did you know?

'Eating for two' Despite the old adage about eating for two during pregnancy, there is actually no need to substantially increase your food intake as your body becomes much more efficient in its use of food and energy when you are pregnant.

Alcohol and caffeine

Every woman knows that excessive alcohol intake is harmful, especially in pregnancy, but few know just how much alcohol might be safe to consume. Similarly, we are increasingly conscious of our caffeine intake, with many of us now drinking decaffeinated beverages.

Alcohol consumption before pregnancy

Many women are unaware of the problems that excessive alcohol intake might cause for the developing baby, and few are aware that alcohol can reduce their fertility. Alcohol can upset the production of eggs from the ovary. A Danish study conducted in 1998 found that women drinking four or fewer units of alcohol a week were twice as likely to conceive than those drinking ten or more units a week. If your partner drinks heavily, this can affect his fertility, too, by upsetting the function of his testicles and their production of both the male hormone testosterone and sperm. However, moderate alcohol intake (up to three or four units a day) does not seem to cause male fertility problems.

The ideal is that you both give up alcohol while you are trying to conceive, or keep your alcohol intake very moderate as no one really knows what is the 'safe' level of alcohol. Remember, too, that if you are trying to get pregnant, you may not know that you have conceived until several weeks after conception, and continued alcohol intake at this point, especially if it is heavy, could harm your developing baby. If you frequently drink heavily and think that you will find it difficult to stop it is worthwhile obtaining specialist advice and counselling before attempting to get pregnant.

Alcohol consumption during pregnancy

During the first two months of pregnancy, the developing baby appears to be particularly vulnerable to the effects of alcohol and it is best to avoid alcohol completely at this time. In particular, avoid binge drinking, where you take a large amount of alcohol over a relatively short period, as the effects of this on the fetus are not yet clear. But if you are usually a light drinker and generally healthy, there appears to be very little chance that if you had too much to drink once early in your pregnancy that it will have harmed your baby.

The only way to be absolutely certain that alcohol does not affect your developing baby is to give it up altogether once you know that you are pregnant and throughout the rest of your pregnancy. Indeed, many women find that they lose the taste for alcohol in pregnancy. This may be the body's natural way of avoiding a potentially toxic substance. However, if you do enjoy the occasional glass of wine, it's worth knowing that there is no confirmed scientific evidence to prove conclusively that drinking under two glasses of wine a day during pregnancy causes a problem.

must know
Alcohol limits
• Generally, it is recommended that, to be on the safe side, you drink no more than two glasses of wine (or its equivalent in alcohol content) once or twice a week.
• Drinking more than 15 glasses of wine a week (or its equivalent) can be associated with a reduction in the baby's birth weight.
• Drinking more than 20 glasses of wine a week can be associated with intellectual impairment in the baby.

Fetal alcohol syndrome

There is no doubt that women who consume large amounts of alcohol in pregnancy can damage their developing baby and extremely high consumption of alcohol on a regular basis can lead to so-called 'fetal alcohol syndrome'. This condition is rare, however, affecting between 1:300 and 1:2,000 pregnancies. The full syndrome affects only about a third of babies whose mothers drink around the equivalent of three bottles of wine a day in pregnancy. The fact that only a third of these babies are affected suggests that other factors such as poor nutrition, genetic make-up or drug abuse need to be present, in addition to heavy alcohol intake, for the syndrome to develop.

Fetal alcohol syndrome has several features: the baby is small; there may be abnormalities in the brain and nervous system that affect development and intellectual ability; there may also be physical abnormalities, such as a short, up-turned nose, receding forehead and chin and asymmetrical ears, causing a characteristic facial deformity.

Coffee consumption before pregnancy

There is no good and consistent evidence that establishes as fact the theory that drinking coffee reduces your fertility. The possibility of an effect has been raised, however, as it has been proposed that caffeine constricts the blood vessels and reduces the blood supply to parts of the body, including the ovaries and the womb, or because it interferes with the metabolism of the female hormone oestrogen.

Remember that caffeine is not only found in coffee. There is caffeine in tea and in some soft drinks like cola.

Coffee consumption during pregnancy

Caffeine crosses the placenta and blood levels in the developing baby are similar to those found in the mother's blood. There is no good evidence to suggest that caffeine ingested in moderate amounts (up to four or five cups a day) harms the developing baby or causes problems, such as miscarriage or premature birth. However, large amounts of caffeine are not recommended in pregnancy as they *might* be associated with problems such as miscarriage, so you should avoid drinking more than five cups of coffee a day. Indeed, it is probably best to avoid taking that much caffeine even if you are not pregnant. Interestingly, many women go off coffee in the first few weeks of pregnancy. This might be the body's own way of limiting caffeine exposure in your developing baby.

must know

Caffeine and smoking
Smoking is known to be linked to impaired growth of the developing baby. When a high caffeine intake is combined with smoking, however, this combination may have a more injurious effect on the baby's growth than the effect of smoking on its own.

Smoking and drugs

Despite our awareness that smoking has a seriously adverse effect on our health, with particular concerns in pregnancy, many young women continue to smoke. They often think they will stop smoking when they conceive. However, smoking does not just affect the development of the baby, but also your ability to conceive successfully.

The effects of smoking

Research has shown that smoking may triple your chances of not being able to conceive. If your partner smokes, he needs to give up as well. Smoking can damage his sperm as well as expose you to passive smoking. However, if you do stop smoking, your fertility returns to normal.

Smoking robs the body of vitamins, especially vitamins B and C, and can cause a build-up of free radicals in the body. Free radicals are molecules that can damage blood vessels, such as those supplying the placenta, thus reducing the supply of nutrients for the developing baby. So smoking is linked to having a small baby as it reduces the ability of the placenta to supply the baby with all the nutrients and oxygen it needs to develop to its full potential. In addition, if you stop smoking, you reduce the risk of certain bleeding problems from the placenta that can complicate the pregnancy and put both you and your baby at risk. Even after pregnancy it is important not to smoke around your baby. This is

watch out!

• Smoking reduces male and female fertility.
• Smoking will reduce your baby's growth.
• While it is best to stop smoking long before conception, stopping during pregnancy will make a difference to your baby and your health. It is never too late to stop.

because the baby will be more prone to 'cot death' and to breathing problems.

All this means that it is important that you stop smoking before becoming pregnant. If your partner is also a smoker, it would be best if you gave up together so that you can support each other. Smoking is a powerful addiction and so it can be very difficult to stop. Your doctor can provide advice or support to help you come off cigarettes or refer you to a smoking cessation programme.

The effects of taking drugs

When planning on getting pregnant or, indeed, if you are pregnant, you should not take street drugs. These are all potentially harmful to your baby. Some, like cocaine, can lead to birth abnormalities; others, such as heroin, methadone, amphetamines and marijuana, can affect the growth of your unborn baby so that it will be small. There is also an increased risk of premature delivery, bleeding from the placenta and an increased risk of infant death. The baby may also suffer from drug withdrawal symptoms after delivery as these drugs cross into the baby's body while it is in the womb. The baby's later development in childhood can also be impaired. In addition, there is a much higher rate of complications to the woman in pregnancy, such as anaemia, infections such as hepatitis and HIV and septicemia from infected needles, and thrombosis (blood clots).

must know

Prescription drugs
Certain drugs or medicines can affect your chances of becoming pregnant and could go on to harm the baby in the womb. Equally, you may require medication for your own continued good health. If you take a pre-scribed medicine on a regular basis, be sure to discuss this with your doctor before you attempt to get pregnant.

Things to avoid

There are some key facts you should know before you conceive as they can sometimes make a big difference to your pregnancy. These range from checking that you are immune to rubella to knowing what foods to avoid that might cause you a problem.

Rubella

Probably better known as German measles, Rubella is a very common infection in children and most children either contract it in childhood or are immunized against it. It is usually a mild condition with a transient rash and swelling of the lymph glands behind the ears. It is caught from airborne droplets that spread when infected people cough or sneeze. German measles, if caught in pregnancy, particularly in the first three months, can cause malformations in your baby. These may include deafness, blindness and heart problems. However, it can only be caught if you are not immune to it, so it is important to know if you are immune to German measles before you try to conceive.

In the UK, children are routinely immunized against German measles, so the vast majority of women are immune. If you're not sure that you have been immunized, your GP should have a record, or your parents may remember. Once you have had rubella or been immunized against it, you should be immune to it. It is rare to lose immunity. If there is any doubt, immunity to German measles can be checked with a simple blood test.

Toxoplasma

Toxoplasma is an organism that usually lives in cats and is found in soil, where it can remain viable for many months.

must know

Immunization before conception
If you are not immune to German measles, you should be immunized before trying to become pregnant. It is then essential to use effective contraception for three months afterwards to avoid getting pregnant. Immunization can not be given during pregnancy as the vaccine is itself a live virus and could cause problems for the baby.

It is excreted in cat feces, so litter trays are potentially a source of infection. Contaminated meat (those most commonly implicated are raw, cured and undercooked meats) and soil-covered vegetables are also a source of infection, so always wash your hands thoroughly after touching soil or raw meat. If gardening, wear rubber gloves.

Recently, it has been found that cats are not the most common source of toxoplasma infection. This may be because cats excrete toxoplasma in their feces only for the first two weeks after they have been infected for the first time. But wear rubber gloves when emptying a cat litter tray as a precaution.

This infection, which can pass from the mother to the developing baby in the womb, has many features in common with congenital rubella. Although it is often asymptomatic in healthy adults, it can sometimes cause particular problems in pregnancy. Toxoplasma infection in adults is usually symptomless or mild, presenting as a mild viral illness. If concerned, your doctor will take a blood test.

Infection of the baby is more likely to occur in later pregnancy, but the risk of damage at this stage is less than in early pregnancy, when it can be a cause of serious abnormalities or lead to miscarriage. However, it is uncommon for babies to be affected in the womb.

• Only about 1–10 out of every 10,000 newborn babies in Europe are infected.

• Overall, about 70 per cent of these infected babies have no associated problem, around ten per cent have eye problems and the remainder have similar problems to those seen with German measles infection (see opposite).

If a toxoplasma infection is suspected in the baby, you will need regular ultrasound examinations and sometimes samples of the baby's blood or amniotic fluid are required to diagnose. The infection can be treated with an antibiotic called spiramycin.

Your weight

It is a fact – young women in the UK are getting heavier. In a little over ten years, the number of women who have a body mass index (see opposite) in the obese range has doubled. While we all know that being very overweight is bad for our health, few women are aware of just how their weight can influence their pregnancy. This is important to know as your weight is something that you can influence before you think about conceiving, and by doing so you make a difference to your health and your pregnancy.

Potential problems associated with weight

If you are trying to conceive and you are seriously overweight or underweight, discuss this with your doctor. Extremes of weight are associated with an increased risk of problems in pregnancy.
• Underweight mothers are more at risk of problems, such as having a small-for-dates baby or going into premature labour.
• Overweight mothers are at risk of problems such as chronic high blood pressure and pre-eclampsia – a serious pregnancy condition related to high blood pressure, which can lead to kidney upset and risk to the baby (see pages 162–3).

In addition, both extremes of weight can be associated with fertility problems (see pages 52–4). You don't want to have to contemplate dieting when you are pregnant (see page 39), so it is important to think about reducing your weight long before trying to get pregnant.

The proportion of people who are overweight in developed countries is increasing. In the UK, around 30 per cent of women are overweight. In the last 10–15 years there has been a doubling in the number of pregnant women who fall into the obese category with their BMI. In the UK today, around 1:5 women who are pregnant are in this obese category and this number is steadily increasing. This is really important as the risk of pregnancy complications is increased in mothers who are obese (see page 52).

Appropriate weight before pregnancy

There is no 'ideal' weight for a woman before pregnancy. Your 'ideal' weight depends on you as an individual and it is not based on what you weigh when you stand on the scales. The way to work out if your pre-pregnancy weight is satisfactory is to calculate your body mass index (BMI), see the box below, and compare the resulting figure with the gradings of BMI given below. This is probably the best guide to weight as it gives a

Calculating your BMI

Your BMI is calculated by taking your body weight in kilograms and dividing it by your height squared (height multiplied by height). For example, if a woman weighs 80 kg (9½ st) and is 1.5 m (4 ft 11 in) tall, her BMI is calculated as follows:

$$\frac{\text{Bodyweight (kg)}}{\text{Height x height (metres)}} = \text{BMI}$$

$\frac{80}{1.5 \times 1.5} = 35.55$, so she would be in the obese category.

However, if this woman had been 1.8 m tall (almost 5 ft 11 in) her BMI would be:

$\frac{80}{1.8 \times 1.8} = 24.69$, which is in the normal BMI category.

Gradings of BMI

Category	Body mass index
Underweight or low	Less than 20
Normal	20.0–25.9
Overweight	26.0–30.9
Obese	31.0–40.9
Extremely obese	41 or more

better indication of body fat content than weight alone, both in pregnant and non-pregnant women. It also takes into account your height, which obviously influences what you should weigh.

The underweight and obese BMI categories are associated with fertility and pregnancy problems. Although it is probably best to be in the normal range before pregnancy, the overweight range is not usually associated with major problems. However, there is some change in the level of risk even in the overweight category. This emphasizes just how important it is to look after your weight.

Body shape
It is not just the quantity of fat you have in your body that matters, but also where it is in your body. Women who are 'pear-shaped', with fat principally on their buttocks and thighs, are at less risk of health problems than those who are 'apple-shaped', carrying fat on their abdomen. Fat in the abdomen influences the metabolism of sugar and fats in your body, with resulting higher levels of sugar and fats in your bloodstream, much more than does fat on your hips. The problems that can be associated with these changes in your metabolism include a risk of pre-eclampsia (see pages 162–3) when you are pregnant and also heart disease in later life. In the last 10 or 15 years it has become clear

The ideal waist circumference for women up to 15 weeks of pregnancy

Ideal	Increased risk	Higher risk
Waist less than 80 cm (31½ in)	Waist 80–87 cm (31½–34 in)	Waist more than 88 cm (34½ in)

that waist circumference is a risk factor for heart disease. Indeed, measuring waist circumference has been advocated as a health-screening test.

• Measure around your waist without any clothes on and do not pull the tape tight; let it lightly rest on the skin.

• Compare the resulting measurement to the table shown opposite.

It has been calculated that a waist circumference of 80 cm (31½ in) or more in early pregnancy almost doubles the risk of high blood pressure and almost triples the risk of pre-eclampsia. Pre-eclampsia is a high blood pressure problem that affects two to three per cent of pregnancies. It causes damage to the blood vessels and can affect not only the mother, but also the baby through damage to the placenta and there are some similarities to the underlying disturbance in blood vessels seen in heart disease.

Other studies suggest that women who have had pre-eclampsia and low-birth weight babies (less than 2.5 kg (5 lb 8 oz)) are more likely to develop heart disease in later life than women who do not develop this complication. If these associations are confirmed, then women who experience these pregnancy complications could benefit from screening after pregnancy for risk factors for heart disease and should seek preventive treatment, including lifestyle modifications, such as better diet and increased exercise. Indeed, there is some evidence to suggest that exercise during early pregnancy (see pages 56–63) or before pregnancy can also reduce the likelihood of pregnancy complications like pre-eclampsia. So getting your waistline into shape before pregnancy, with a good diet and regular exercise, might not only be good for your figure but also for the health of you and your baby.

Pregnancy risks for the overweight mother

Your pre-pregnancy weight has the biggest effect on your baby's birth weight and is a more important factor than weight gain in pregnancy (see pages 54-5). Women who are very overweight, particularly those with a BMI over 30 when they embark on pregnancy, have an increased risk of problems (see pages 48-9).

Additional tests for overweight pregnant women

- Your doctor may offer you an additional ultrasound scan at around 18-20 weeks to check for fetal abnormality.
- You may also be checked for pregnancy-induced diabetes. This requires a test in which you take a glucose drink after an overnight fast. Your blood sugar is checked before and after the glucose drink.
- You are also checked regularly for the complications that are more common in overweight mothers, such as pre-eclampsia. Sometimes you will require treatment to prevent a thrombosis from occurring – your doctor will advise you about this.
- Your weight is checked at regular intervals throughout the pregnancy.

Labour and delivery risks

Slow progress in labour is more common if you are very overweight, so you will have a higher chance of having a Caesarean delivery. Emergency Caesarean carries a higher risk of complications than a planned one performed before labour, especially if you are very overweight. Sometimes a planned Caesarean section is considered the least hazardous mode of delivery. The plan for your delivery must be suited to your own particular situation and needs, however, and you should discuss this with your doctor, who is able to give you the specific advice required. If you are having a normal vaginal delivery and the baby is large, the doctors and midwives watch for shoulder dystocia, in which the size of the baby's shoulders can cause difficulty in delivery.

After delivery, an overweight mother is also likely to need treatment to prevent blood clots, often with injections of heparin under the skin, especially if the baby was delivered by Caesarean section. Women who are overweight are more likely to get infections, such as an infection in their caesarean section wound or a urinary tract infection, which is usually associated with pain on passing urine.

While breastfeeding is being established, it is best to avoid dieting as this can affect your milk production. However, once feeding is established, you can lose up to 2 kg (4½ lb) each month.

Losing weight before pregnancy

Strict dieting to lose a lot of weight is not advisable either when trying to get pregnant or during pregnancy. This is because you may disturb your nutritional balance at crucial stages of your baby's development. But for women in the overweight and obese BMI ranges, substantial health benefits can be obtained by even modest reductions in weight.

Outside of pregnancy it has been estimated that losing 10 kg (around 22 lb) results in a ten per cent fall in cholesterol, and a significant reduction in blood pressure. In pregnancy, a woman with a BMI in the overweight range above 25 doubles her risk of pre-eclampsia, while if she has a BMI in the obese category (greater than 30), she has at least a three-fold increase in

must know

Weight considerations for assisted conception treatment
If a woman is overweight the success of assisted conception is reduced so she should take her BMI into account. This is a very sensible measure for a number of reasons:
• women who are very overweight have reduced fertility
• losing weight can increase fertility
• carrying out assisted conception treatment is technically difficult for women who are very overweight
• the success rate is substantially lower. Women with a BMI greater than 30 have a 30 per cent lower success rate with IVF

must know

Take exercise
Exercise plays an important part when trying to lose weight. Your weight depends on the balance between the food you take in and the energy you burn up. If you take in more energy from your food than you burn up with exercise, you will gain weight. If you do not take much regular exercise, build up the amount gradually before you get pregnant (see pages 56–63).

risk. But perhaps the greatest effect can be seen with the risk of getting gestational diabetes. Compared with a woman with a BMI of 20–25, a woman with a BMI of 26–29 has just over a three-fold increase in the risk of having diabetes in pregnancy, but if her BMI is over 30, the risk is more than 15 times higher. So the risks of many of these complications, including birth defects, is related directly to BMI. The higher the BMI, the higher the risk, so if you have an increased BMI any reduction in weight you can make pre-pregnancy is valuable.

Ideally, specialist advice is required to provide you with an individualized assessment and management plan. Specific help from dietitian and support groups is invaluable in losing weight and maintaining it. It is also valuable to consult your doctor for a full health assessment to help identify any additional or associated problems, like high blood pressure or high blood lipids (fats), which might need specific treatment.

When losing weight, set a realistic target over a period of around three months. Then, in the longer term, to maintain a steady weight and avoid further increases, aim to establish a change in your diet and exercise patterns.

As you correct your weight, you may start to ovulate and so fall pregnant when you were not expecting it. This might be before you and your body are ready for it. Because of this, you might want to consider using contraception until you have reached your target weight.

Weight gain during pregnancy

Your weight, of course, increases in pregnancy, but only a small amount of this weight gain is fat. Unless you are very underweight or overweight, doctors are not too concerned about weight gain in pregnancy. This is because the growth of the baby is not dependent on your weight gain, but rather upon the efficiency of transfer of vital nutrients across the placenta. However, on average, women gain around 12 kg (26 lb) during pregnancy. Some women gain less and some more, depending on several factors, including how heavy you are to start with and how big your baby is.

Of the 12 kg (26 lb) weight gain in an 'average' pregnancy, most of this is made up by the womb, baby, placenta and amniotic fluid, which by full term weighs almost 6 kg (13 lb) in total. Extra fat and the increased weight of your breasts account for 3.9 kg (8 lb 7 oz) of the weight gain, while the rest is made up of an increase in the volume of your blood and by retained fluid.

These estimates vary enormously from woman to woman and the figures given below are simply an illustration of how the weight gain is made up. Remember that the fat that you gain in pregnancy is there for a reason. Your body is deliberately storing fat on your hips, your back and your breasts to prepare you for breastfeeding. Milk is rich in fats, which are needed by the growing baby. Not surprisingly, women who breastfeed lose weight faster after pregnancy than those who do not.

did you know?

Limiting weight gain

Keeping the amount of weight gain in pregnancy low is important for women who are seriously over-weight as this reduces the risk of pregnancy complications, such as high blood pressure or having a very large baby. Even if you put on no weight in pregnancy, this does not affect the baby, provided you have a balanced diet. Discuss this with your doctor, who can give you specific advice.

What weight gain in pregnancy typically might consist of

Baby	3.5 kg (7 lb 8 oz)
Placenta	0.5 kg (1 lb 2 oz)
Amniotic fluid	0.8 kg (1 lb 12 oz)
Increase in weight of the womb	0.7 kg (1 lb 8 oz)
Breasts	0.4 kg (14 oz)
Blood volume	1.3 kg (2 lb 9 oz)
Fat	3.5 kg (7 lb 8 oz)
Fluid retention	1.3 kg (2 lb 9 oz)

Exercise during pregnancy

Just as with diet, exercise is critical to good health. Both combine to influence our weight. Food is our fuel. If we don't burn it off with exercise, we store it as fat. To maintain a steady body weight, food supply should be balanced with energy expenditure.

Exercise is good

Pre-pregnancy most women know that exercise is good for their health. Many women are concerned, however, that they may have to stop exercising in pregnancy as this might threaten the pregnancy. In general, this is not true and exercise is encouraged during pregnancy.

There is extensive research to show that, in most cases, exercise is safe for both mother and baby. Doctors therefore recommend initiating or continuing exercise in pregnancy because of the health benefits. Indeed, athletes who continue training in pregnancy actually have an improved performance after the pregnancy as the pregnancy-induced changes in the cardiovascular system enhance the effect of training. Not only does regular exercise make you feel better and fitter, it also helps prepare you physically for labour and delivery.

Walking, cycling, swimming and stretching are all good forms of exercise in pregnancy. However, you should avoid activities that are likely to lead to any falls or impacts on your abdomen, such as contact sports like kick boxing. In later pregnancy, activities where balance is important, such as horse riding or down-hill skiing, can be hazardous due to the change in your centre of gravity.

• Swimming is a particularly good form of exercise when you are pregnant. This is because the water supports your body and you can exercise your arms, legs and back and also improve cardiovascular fitness without straining your body.

• Yoga is also a good form of exercise and an ideal preparation for labour because of the muscular stretching, control of breathing and posture, and emphasis on relaxation.

So for most women, the exercises they have been doing pre-pregnancy can be continued. For those who have not been taking regular exercise, it is worth thinking seriously about starting a routine during pregnancy.

The important thing about taking exercise is to do it regularly. Thirty minutes of moderate exercise three times a week or more makes a big difference to your fitness and your weight. You should also increase your exercise as you go about your daily activities. Walk wherever possible and take the stairs instead of the lift. Regular exercise is also good for reducing stress and makes you feel more energetic, as well as increasing your sense of wellbeing.

Benefits of exercise in pregnancy

- greater feeling of wellbeing and less tiredness
- may help reduce feelings of stress and anxiety
- less lower back pain
- less likelihood of varicose veins
- may reduce the risk of certain pregnancy complications, such as diabetes and blood pressure problems
- prepares you for the physical demands of labour
- may have a shorter labour

Beginning to take exercise

If you are not used to regular exercise, start gradually with a low-intensity, low-impact activity like swimming or walking. Begin with a good 15 minutes of aerobic exercise, like walking or swimming three times weekly, and build up to about 30 minutes three or four times a week, and then every day. A brisk 30 minutes of walking, ideally with part of it up hill, three times a week, leads to improvements in fitness within two weeks. This builds up your stamina, which is one of the major objectives of exercising in pregnancy.

Key points to remember when taking exercise are:
- aerobics (exercise that improve the fitness of your cardiovascular system) and strength-conditioning exercises are recommended for pregnancy health, aiming for a good level of fitness rather than peak competitive athletic performance
- appropriate levels of exercise are not linked to pregnancy complications and, in fact, might reduce the risk of certain complications
- after delivery, moderate exercise does not affect breastfeeding in any way.

Before you start each exercise session, it is worth spending four to five minutes on muscle warm-ups. A 'cool down' period of gradually declining exercise at the end of the session is also advisable. It is usually best to limit your activity to 15-minute periods with five minutes of rest in between.

Ideally you will have an individual fitness programme that takes into account your age, level of fitness and any other relevant factor, such as a pre-existing medical condition. The target heart rates for aerobic exercise in pregnancy are shown in

watch out!
- If you have any medical or obstetric problems, consult your doctor before starting any exercise programme.
- If you have any unusual symptoms when exercising, stop and obtain advice from your doctor.
- Stop exercising if you feel very short of breath, get chest pain, feel faint or dizzy, have a bad headache, or have any vaginal bleeding, or leg swelling, or abdominal pain and seek your doctor's advice.

Mother's age (years)	Maximum heart rate target per minute
Less than 20	140–155
20–30	135–150
30 – 40	130–145
Over 40	125–140

the table above, but if you are not used to exercise, you should set a target about 60 per cent above your usual heart rate. So, if your usual rate is about 80, a suitable maximum would be about 125 beats per minute.

Exercise to avoid

You should avoid prolonged, high-intensity training and the general rule for exercise is to not overdo it when you are pregnant. If you are too breathless to hold a conversation when exercising, then you are probably doing too much.

• Check your heart rate (see table, above) and don't exceed your target rate.

• Do not get overheated or dehydrated; in particular, do not exercise if you have a high temperature.

• Do not exercise for prolonged periods; do no more than 45 minutes at a time.

• Ensure that you always have a good fluid intake after vigorous exercise.

In terms of what exercises to do regularly, avoid sit-ups and straight leg raising while on your back. These can strain your abdominal muscles, which are already stretched by the growing pregnancy. The two large muscles that run longitudinally down the middle of your abdomen (known collectively as the rectus abdominus), normally separate in pregnancy to help accommodate the growing pregnancy. Exercises that stretch these muscles, such as sit-ups and straight leg raising, stresses them further, which slows down the speed at which they return to normal after the pregnancy.

In addition, when you get up from lying down, take care not to strain the abdominal muscles. Roll over on to your side, push yourself up with your arms, then get into a kneeling position and stand up, one leg at a time while keeping your back straight.

Another reason not to exercise while lying on your back in pregnancy is to avoid feeling faint. When you are pregnant and lie on your back, the weight of the pregnancy can obstruct the large blood vessels in your abdomen that are pumping the blood back to the heart. The heart therefore has less blood to pump out and so you can feel faint.

If you feel any strain during exercise, stop at once to prevent damage to your ligaments. Your ligaments are very strong fibrous bands of tissue that hold bones together, including those of the pelvis and they soften in pregnancy to allow more room in the pelvis to help ease the passage of the baby through the birth canal. However, this softening also makes them more likely to be strained if you stretch too far.

Jogging
From 20 weeks onwards, it is thought best by some doctors to avoid exercises that cause the womb and the baby to bounce up and down on your pelvic floor (such as jogging and jumping) because this might lead to weakening of your pelvic floor. However,

other doctors believe that moderate amounts of jogging are not harmful.

Jogging can stress your joints and your breasts, so if you do jog, wear a supportive sport's bra and running shoes that absorb some of the shock. If you are a serious runner and jog frequently, it is probably best to reduce the number of kilometres you do after 28 weeks of pregnancy, and further reduce it after 36 weeks. This is because there is some concern that strenuous prolonged exercise at this stage of pregnancy could reduce the blood supply to the baby. You can, of course, replace jogging with less strenuous forms of exercise in later pregnancy.

When exercise is best avoided

You should avoid vigorous or strenuous exercise in certain situations, and in other conditions more care and supervision may be required (see table, below). If you have a medical problem, talk to your doctor about exercise before you embark on a routine before or during pregnancy. It is sometimes best to restrict yourself to stretching-type exercises only.

Conditions where strenuous exercise should be avoided (check with your doctor)	Conditions where strenuous exercise in pregnancy needs more care and supervision (check with your doctor)
• Significant heart disease	• Diabetes
• Recurrent miscarriage, particularly due to cervical incompetence (see pages 154–5)	• High blood pressure
• Premature labour	• Anaemia
• Ruptured membranes	• Twin pregnancies
• Vaginal bleeding in pregnancy	• Extreme obesity
• A small-for-dates baby	

Using a sauna or hot tub after exercise

It is best to avoid a sauna or hot tub as the risk of getting overheated is more likely in pregnancy, especially after exercise, which can make you faint. If you do have a sauna, limit the time to no longer than five minutes and also limit the temperature to less than 82 °C (179.6 °F). If you have a hot tub, limit the time to a maximum of 15 minutes at a temperature of less than 39 °C (102.2 °F). If you feel uncomfortable or faint, get out immediately. You should also make sure that you maintain your fluid intake as the heat can be very dehydrating.

Pelvic floor exercises

The pelvic floor is a sheet of muscle and fibrous tissue lying across the bottom of the pelvis. It supports the pelvic organs, including the bladder, part of the bowel and the womb, while the vagina, bowel and urethra (the tube that takes urine from the bladder to the outside) pass through it. The pelvic floor therefore helps you keep control of your bladder and bowel function. When you want to stop passing urine mid-stream, it is the pelvic floor muscles that you contract to do so.

These muscles can be stretched and damaged by the stress of pregnancy and delivery, which can lead to problems such as stress incontinence, where increased pressure on the pelvic floor, such as with coughing, leads to a small leak of urine from the

watch out!

Other activities that are best to avoid when pregnant include:
• any activity like horseriding that might be associated with loss of balance or trauma to the developing baby
• any exercising at high altitudes, such as skiing in the mountains, as there is less oxygen at high altitudes, which in turn might lead to a reduced oxygen supply for the baby
• scuba diving, because of the possible effects of decompression sickness on the baby, which are potentially dangerous

bladder. It thus makes sense to strengthen the pelvic floor before and during pregnancy to minimize the risk of problems later on. Pelvic floor exercises are designed to do this and should be performed both during and after pregnancy.

Raising the pelvic floor

First, pull up and tense the muscles around your urethra, vagina and rectum as if you are interrupting the flow of urine. Hold for several seconds, then release and relax. Repeat four to five times and then repeat this set ten times and thereafter several times a day. You may want to try fitting these exercises into your daily routine, so try practising them each time you pass urine.

Avoiding back strain

The increased load on your body from the growing pregnancy often leads to backache. You need to think about your posture and avoid stooping or slumping forward as this stresses your back more. When you are sitting, tuck a cushion behind the lower part of your back to help you sit up straight. You should avoid exercises and activities that might strain your back. Do not do any heavy lifting or load bearing as this can also strain your back. If you have to lift something heavy, like a young child, bend your legs to get down, keep your back straight and lift by straightening your legs. Keep the child close to your body as lifting something at arms' length can add to the strain on your back.

3 Fertility problems and treatment

Fertility problems are common: 1:6 couples are affected. However, the last 25 years has seen an explosion in our knowledge of male and female fertility and our technical ability to treat a whole range of fertility problems. So it is important to know that if you do have a problem, there is now a great deal that can be done to help you conceive.

Conception difficulties

When a couple have difficulty conceiving, it is often thought to be the woman's problem. This is a misconception and so it is important to take the couple into consideration rather than the man or the woman individually.

Potential reasons for conception difficulties

• In a third of cases, there is a problem with sperm quantity or quality.

• In around a quarter of cases, there may be a problem in producing eggs.

• In a fifth of cases, problems with the fallopian tubes prevent transport of the eggs to the womb.

Furthermore, it is not uncommon for more than one factor to be present and in almost 1:5 couples, both partners contribute to the problem. However, in about a quarter of cases, no cause can be found in either partner. This is called unexplained infertility (see page 85). In addition, the problem can be something that you might not consider to be a medical issue, like being underweight or overweight, experiencing rapid weight loss or smoking.

What is 'infertility'?

Humans are not highly efficient when it comes to fertility. About 20 per cent of couples will conceive within a month of beginning to try, rising to 70 per cent within six months. After a year of regular unprotected intercourse only around 84 per cent of normal fertile couples will have conceived. In those couples who have not conceived after a year, around half of those continuing to try to conceive will succeed within a further twelve months. So do not be alarmed if you do not get pregnant within the first few months of trying for a baby. Infertility is usually defined as an inability to conceive after a minimum of twelve months of unprotected intercourse. Doctors do not usually investigate for a fertility problem unless you had been trying unsuccessfully for at least a year. This is because many 'normal' couples take at least this long to conceive.

• Primary infertility is a term used to describe couples who are having difficulty in conceiving and who have not previously had a pregnancy.

• Secondary infertility is used to describe couples who have previously had a pregnancy but subsequently found they have difficulty conceiving. This applies even if the first pregnancy was not successful. For example, a woman who has had several miscarriages and then has difficulty conceiving again has secondary infertility.

So even if you have had a pregnancy in the past, you may still have difficulty conceiving. When this happens, you should consider whether there have been any changes since your pregnancy. For example:

• has one of you developed a medical problem since the previous pregnancy? This could be something such as an operation for appendicitis (see page 70) in the woman or treatment for testicular cancer in the man

• have you formed a new relationship and so have a different partner since your previous pregnancy?

• has it been a long time since the previous pregnancy such that you are now a lot older than you were when you last conceived? Doctors know that fertility declines in a woman as she gets older, particularly after the age of 35 years.

must know
Conception facts
• Around 16 per cent of couples have some difficulty conceiving.
• About 20 per cent of couples conceive within a month, rising to 70 per cent within six months.
• Only around 84 per cent of normal fertile couples conceive within a year of regular unprotected intercourse.
• In those couples who have not conceived after a year, around half of those continuing to try to conceive succeed within a further twelve months.
• Therefore, after two years of unprotected intercourse, around 92 per cent of couples have conceived.

The main fertility problems in women

- The ovaries may not produce or release an egg every month.
- The fallopian tubes that carry the egg from the ovary down to the womb may be blocked. This blockage prevents the fertilized egg reaching the womb or even being fertilized, as the sperm meets the egg in the fallopian tube.
- Endometriosis can also cause damage to the tubes and ovaries. This is a condition where tissue similar to the lining of the womb grows on places such as the ovary, the tube or in the pelvis. Every month this tissue passes through a cycle, just as the lining of the womb, but, there is no way for the blood to escape and this leads to inflammation and scarring.
- Sometimes, the lining of the womb may not be ready for the implantation of a fertilized egg.
- There can be difficulty in the sperm getting from the vagina to the womb. This is because the mucous, which is at the neck of the womb, may be too thick or hostile to the sperm, preventing them from passing through the mucous at the cervix and into the womb itself.
- Age. Fertility wanes after the age of 35 years and especially after a woman passes 40. For example, only 77 per cent of fertile 38-year-old women conceive after three years of unprotected intercourse. Older women are likely to not only produce fewer eggs, but the eggs they do produce may not be so able to implant into the womb after fertilization as they were at a younger age. Age has much less of an effect on male fertility.

Lack of egg production

A common cause for a woman having difficulty conceiving is a hormonal imbalance that upsets the

must know
Causes of endometriosis

Doctors don't really know why endometriosis occurs. It may result from fragments of the tissue lining the womb (endometrium) 'escaping' down the fallopian tube and into the abdomen during a menstrual period. These fragments then 'seed' onto the tissues in the abdomen and patches of endometriosis form. These patches behave as though they were in the womb, producing a 'period' each month. The endometriosis tissue needs the female hormone oestrogen to survive, so endometriosis is not found in girls before puberty or in women after the menopause when oestrogen levels are very low.

process of egg production or ovulation every month. Polycystic ovary syndrome (PCOS) is one of the most common disorders that upset ovulation. This is considered the major reason for women not producing an egg every month. If you have PCOS, the symptoms you are likely to experience are irregular, very spaced out or even absent periods, a greasier skin and acne and excess body hair. These three features do not always occur together. In this condition, an egg starts to develop every month, but because the hormone levels that control egg production are imbalanced, the egg stops maturating and is left as a tiny follicle or 'cyst' on the ovary. These are not true cysts on the ovary but rather small follicles where an egg has started to develop but stops before it matures (see page 8).

Other medical problems, like thyroid disease, can also affect production of the egg. If you are very overweight with a BMI of over 29 (see page 49), this can also upset the ability of your ovaries to produce an egg every month because excess fat can cause a hormonal imbalance. This can be improved simply by losing weight, which often leads not only to a more regular menstrual cycle but also better fertility. Even a modest amount of weight loss in this situation can make a big difference. Women who are very underweight may also have a disturbance in their menstrual cycle. In this situation, weight gain makes a difference. For more information on weight, see pages 48–55.

Fallopian tube blockage
The fallopian tubes can be blocked by an infection, such as a sexually transmitted disease, which can cause scarring of the tube and so prevent the sperm and the egg meeting. In the worst cases both tubes can be

must know

Fibroids

A fibroid is a benign lump of muscle in your womb and although fibroids can sometimes cause your periods to be heavy simply because they make the womb bigger so that there is more lining to shed each time you have a period, it is unusual for fibroids to affect your fertility. Very occasionally the womb can become so distorted by a large fibroid or multiple fibroids that this can lead to recurrent mis-carriages, but such cases are usually not common.

blocked. Previous surgery in the abdomen can also cause scarring to the tube. One of the most common causes of this would be surgery for appendicitis. With appendicitis there is a significant amount of inflammation within the pelvis and that, plus the surgery itself, can irritate the tissues and cause problems, such as adhesions around the fallopian tube, and so lead to a blockage. Damage to a tube can also occur after an ectopic pregnancy, which often requires all or part of the tube to be removed completely.

Endometriosis

Endometriosis is a condition where tissue similar to the tissue found in the lining of the womb (endometrium) occurs in small patches in sites outside the womb. It can sometimes be found in the muscle of the womb, when it is termed adenomyosis. The most common sites are on the ovaries, fallopian tubes and the ligaments in the pelvis that support the womb. Often it produces no symptoms, but sometimes it can cause problems because each month, when a period occurs, the small patches of endometriosis also bleed. The blood cannot escape from the body and it irritates and inflames the surrounding tissues, causing pain. Chronic irritation of the tissues can lead to scarring and adhesions in the pelvis where tissues stick together. This can sometimes cause problems with a woman's fertility due to the tubes being obstructed by adhesions or the ovaries being caught up with adhesions, preventing release of the egg. The main symptoms of endometriosis are pain in the abdomen and pelvis, pain when a woman is on her period (dysmenorrhea) and pain experienced deep in the pelvis during intercourse.

Endometriosis can sometimes cause infertility. If you have severe endometriosis, with damage to the fallopian tubes or where your ovaries are trapped in adhesions preventing release of the egg, this obviously reduces your fertility. Doctors are uncertain whether mild endometriosis, where the tubes and ovaries remain normal, actually causes infertility. However, it is certainly more common in women with infertility. Indeed around 30 per cent of those with endometriosis have a fertility problem.

Female anatomy.

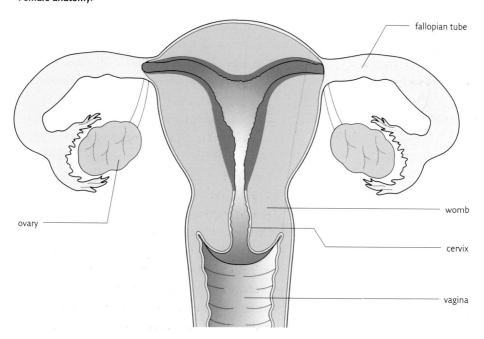

fallopian tube

ovary

womb

cervix

vagina

The lining of the womb

The fertilized egg implants into the lining of the womb. Doctors still do not fully understand just how this critical event occurs, but they do know that if the lining of the womb (the endometrium) is not ready for the fertilized egg, that implantation may fail. This lack of preparation might be due to insufficient progesterone, the hormone that prepares the lining of the womb for implantation, or it might be because the lining of the womb does not respond to the progesterone. This can be found in somewhere between 3 and 20 per cent of couples with a fertility problem. However, much of this information is not consistent and at present there is no good evidence that treatment can improve this. Furthermore, its role as a cause of infertility has been questioned. Doctors therefore do not routinely check the lining of the womb to evaluate its suitability for implantation.

Thickened or hostile mucous

Doctors know that some cases of infertility might be linked to 'hostile' cervical mucus, which the sperm finds difficult to penetrate and so cannot reach the womb. Many of the current treatments of fertility problems circumvent the sperm passing through the mucus by using assisted conception techniques.

The main fertility problems in men

● If a man does not produce enough sperm or the sperm are of poor quality, this can lead to difficulty in conceiving.

● There can sometimes be difficulty in the sperm travelling from the testicles down the fine tubes that carry the sperm to the penis (see page 17).

Sometimes these tubes can be blocked and so, even though enough sperm is produced, it cannot reach the vagina or the fallopian tube to fertilize the egg that is waiting.

• Men who have an undescended testicle, which is often treated by surgery in childhood, may have a problem producing sufficient sperm, as can those who have surgery in the area of the testicle, including a hernia repair.

• The testicles are outside the body for a reason. Sperm production occurs best at a slightly lower temperature than your body. So there is a link between tight clothing and increased temperature of the scrotum that might impact on sperm production. Doctors are not certain whether wearing loose fitting underwear actually makes a difference and improves the quality of sperm, but it seems like a reasonable and simple thing to think about doing if you have a low sperm count.

• Sometimes, a viral infection like mumps when you are an adult can affect the testicles and lead to a problem in sperm production.

• Difficulties in sperm production can sometimes be caused by genetic problems.

• Certain medications for medical conditions can have an impact, too. In particular, both radiotherapy and chemotherapy for cancer treatment can cause difficulties with male fertility.

• Infections, including sexually transmitted infections, can cause scarring and blockage of the fine tubes that allow the sperm to travel from the testicles to the penis.

• Just as with women, if a man is overweight with a BMI over 29 (see page 49) his fertility can be impaired.

Seeking help

If you have been trying for a baby for more than a year, it is time to seek medical advice. Ideally, you and your partner should see the doctor together, rather than separately.

Consulting your doctor

The doctor will take a detailed history from you both, including your age, how long you have been trying to conceive, how often you have intercourse, previous contraception, whether you have any problems with intercourse, the presence of chronic medical conditions or long-term medication, and details of any previous pregnancies (including any pregnancies with previous partners and also any terminations of pregnancy).

You will be asked about menstrual problems and any history of pelvic infection or abdominal surgery. This is because infection or abdominal operations can lead to problems such as adhesions, which can cause the fallopian tubes to be blocked. Your partner will be asked about his occupation, any past medical problems, surgical operations or trauma to the testicles and any infections that can affect the genitals, such as mumps in adulthood. He will also be asked about any regular medication (as this can sometimes upset sperm function) and about any sexual difficulty such as premature ejaculation. The doctor will also want to know if either of you smoke and how much alcohol you drink. This is because smoking can reduce your fertility and excess alcohol consumption can upset sperm quality. You both may be examined.

Initial investigations

Your doctor will tell you if there are any obvious problems and whether a specialist referral is required. Your doctor will give you some general advice, and point out the most important issues, such as the need to take folic acid, stop smoking, cut down or stop drinking alcohol, and you will be asked about your immunity to rubella and whether your cervical smear tests are up to date. You may also be checked for anaemia and hepatitis or HIV, as testing is needed prior to assisted conception because these conditions may have implications for the baby. If your doctor suspects you have endometriosis, you will be referred on for visual identification of the tissue.

If you are overweight, your doctor will advise about the need to reduce weight or limit weight gain (see pages 48–55). It is unlikely that you will be asked to use temperature charts or ovulation prediction kits in the first instance (see pages 13–15) as there is little evidence to show that they improve success over regular intercourse occurring every couple of days throughout the cycle. If you have a particular medical problem, such as diabetes or heart disease, specialist referral may be required to obtain advice about the effect of this condition on any pregnancy and also the effect of pregnancy on your condition.

did you know?
Seeking help early
In some situations, you might want to seek an earlier assessment of your fertility. If, for example, there is a known factor that might affect fertility in you or your partner, such as an undescended testicle, cancer therapy, very irregular or absent periods, damage to the fallopian tubes from surgery or infection, or if the women is aged over 35 years.

did you know?

Non-steroidal anti-inflammatory drugs (NSAIDS)
These are used commonly for the treatment of pain, inflammation and fever and can upset ovulation. They interfere with the synthesis of chemical messengers important for the release of the mature egg. So, although the menstrual cycle seems normal and an egg is produced, it is not released. Women who use these medications on a regular basis, such as for chronic arthritis, may encounter difficulty conceiving and stopping the medication may solve the problem.

More specialized assessments

Your initial investigations can be performed by a GP, but more detailed assessment and treatment requires referral to a specialist. There are three key questions, ordered by ease of testing, that will need to be answered:

• do you produce an egg (ovulate) regularly?
• is your partner's sperm production satisfactory?
• is there any problem with your fallopian tubes that could prevent transport of the egg?

Assessing ovulation

If you have regular periods with a cycle of 21–35 days, this suggests that you are ovulating regularly. If you experience Mittelschmerz (mid-cycle pain associated with ovulation), changes in your cervical mucous and increased temperature mid-cycle, these features also suggest that you are ovulating (see pages 8–15). However, to be sure that you are ovulating, the key medical investigation is to measure the concentration of progesterone in a blood sample taken seven days before your expected period is due. If you have an irregular cycle, then several samples may be required, each taken a few days apart. Progesterone is only produced in high quantities after ovulation, so a high progesterone level means that you have ovulated. If you are not ovulating, then further hormonal assessments will be required to identify the cause.

Assessing sperm problems

Your partner will be asked to produce a semen sample through masturbation after abstaining from intercourse for at least two days. You should not collect the sample in a condom – most condoms have spermicidal lubricants that make analysis impossible. Nor should the sample be collected by coitus interruptus (withdrawal during intercourse) as much of the sample can be lost – remember that some semen is often released prior to ejaculation proper, which you may not be aware of. Instead, collect the sample in a wide-mouthed plastic specimen pot and promptly transport it to the laboratory, avoiding extremes of temperature. As there is marked variation in semen from day to day and week to week, at least two specimens should be assessed.

A normal semen sample has a volume of 2–4 ml (½–1 tsp) with more than 20 million sperm in each millilitre and a total of at least 40 million sperm in an ejaculate. At least 50 per cent of the sperm cells should be able to move forward, 75 per cent should be live, and more than 15 per cent of the sperm cells should have a normal form. If the analysis suggests

did you know?

Further tests
If you have an irregular cycle or infrequent periods, you will be offered additional tests on the hormones controlling egg production and release to look for an underlying disturbance in the key hormones. If you have symptoms that might be indicative of a thyroid problem (see page 182-4), then your thyroid gland function will also be checked.

a sperm problem, the test should be repeated. As it takes around 70 days for sperm to mature, it is usual to allow two to three months between samples so that any temporary upset in sperm production will be rectified. If there is a more extreme problem, such as no sperm in the ejaculate, then the test is repeated as soon as possible.

Assessing the function of the fallopian tubes

Several investigative methods are available for assessing tubal function. X-ray assessment of the tubes is commonly used. Special dye that appears white on an X-ray is injected through the cervix. An X-ray is then taken and the outline of the womb and tubes will be seen. If the dye is seen spilling into the abdomen, then the tubes are open. This test will also check if the womb is normally shaped. Ultrasound can also be used in a similar way to determine if your tubes are open. However, you should know that even if the tubes are open they may not necessarily function normally. For example, the lining of the tube may have been damaged by infection in the past, so preventing normal transport of the egg down the tube to the womb.

If there is the possibility that you have endometriosis as well as a fertility problem, then diagnostic laparoscopy is considered by many gynaecologists as the method of choice. During the procedure, which usually requires general anaesthesia, a laparoscope (a telescope-like instrument) is inserted into the abdomen through a small cut, usually below the navel, so that the surgeon can view and assess the womb, fallopian tubes and ovaries. Blue dye is injected through the cervix using an instrument placed in the cervix through the vagina. The dye flows through the womb and fallopian tubes and, if the tubes are open, spills into the abdomen. Through the laparoscope, patches of endometriosis appear like blue or black spots and sometimes scar tissue and adhesions are seen.

As infection is the most common cause of tubal damage. Your doctor may suggest a test to look for evidence of past or current infection that might be affecting the tubes.

Womb with endometriosis on the ovary.

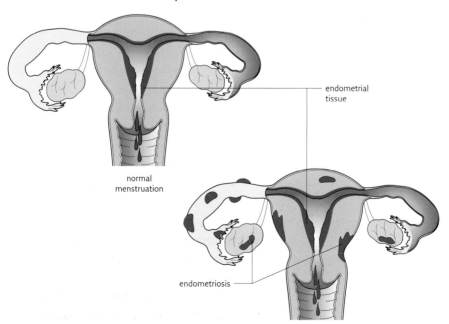

endometrial tissue

normal menstruation

endometriosis

Fertility treatments

As you have seen, many couples have fertility problems, but this does not mean that they cannot have a baby. There is now the potential for the vast majority of fertility problems to be treated and success rates are good. So if you have a problem, the outlook is usually optimistic. Some fertility problems can be treated without recourse to assisted conception techniques and it is these treatments that this section is concerned with.

Treating a disturbance in ovulation

The treatment of disturbance of ovulation depends on the reason causing the disturbance. Irregular or infrequent periods are most commonly due to a hormonal disturbance affecting the ability of the ovaries to produce eggs. Sometimes the cause is not directly linked to the hormones controlling the ovaries, but to other hormones that have a knock-on effect. For example, upsets in your thyroid or adrenal glands can also disturb ovarian function. Obviously, if you have a specific problem, such as thyroid disease, or you don't produce the hormones that regulate the ovary this should be treated directly. Your specialist will be able to advise you on the best treatment for your particular problem.

Correcting an excess of prolactin

One such problem is an excess of the hormone prolactin. This hormone, produced from the pituitary gland at the base of the brain, stimulates milk production after pregnancy, but sometimes women can produce high levels of this when they are not pregnant. This hormone not only stimulates milk production but inhibits egg production.

This means that women who are exclusively breastfeeding don't ovulate regularly until their baby is weaned. However, if you develop high levels of this hormone when you are not pregnant, your periods will become infrequent, ovulation will be disturbed and you may notice some milk leaking from your nipples. This can be treated with a medication, such as bromocriptine, which suppresses the prolactin production and allows ovulation to occur.

Ovulation induction through medication

Most commonly it is a disturbance in the balance of hormones controlling the ovaries that causes irregular ovulation and this can be treated with medication, usually clomifene. Clomifene is given in tablet form and the medication enhances the body's normal hormonal changes that lead to egg production – known as ovulation induction. Some side effects of clomifene are hot flushes, nausea and breast tenderness. Its success is checked by measuring progesterone levels in the blood.

One drawback of this therapy, however, is that sometimes the ovaries produce more than one egg in response to stimulation so that there is an increased risk of conceiving twins or even triplets. Where this is considered a significant risk, the response of the ovaries to the drugs is monitored through regular blood hormone measurement or ultrasound to visualize the eggs developing on the ovaries. These checks may only be needed during the first cycle of treatment so that your response to this medication can be assessed.

If you are overweight with a BMI of more than 25 and don't respond to medication like clomifene, then metformin may be added to the clomifene treatment to improve the response. This medication can sometimes cause some nausea and gastric upset.

must know
Clomifene and IVF
This tablet form of ovulation induction is not suitable for linking in with procedures like IVF (see pages 94–7).

It is often useful to combine these ovulation induction treatments with intrauterine insemination, where your partner's sperm is injected directly into the womb (see pages 100–01).

Hormone injections

If there is no response to a medication such as clomifene, hormone injections can be used, which are more powerful. The risk of twins or triplets is relatively high with this treatment. This technique is usually used in in vitro fertilization (IVF) (see pages 94–7).

Ovarian drilling

This is a surgical treatment that occurs at the time of laparoscopy and small holes are drilled in the surface of the ovary. The treatment seems to make the ovary more likely to produce eggs.

Treating a low sperm count

In cases where there is no sperm in the seminal fluid, the task is to determine whether there is a problem with production or whether the tubes connecting the testicles to the penis are blocked. Blockage can be treated surgically. If absolutely no sperm is being produced, this implies a problem with the testicles or hormones controlling sperm production and specialist help is required, such as hormone treatment. However, this can only help if the cause is a deficiency in the hormones that control sperm production and the male hormone testosterone.

It is rare for a man to have absolutely no sperm. More commonly, the sperm count will be low or there will be reduced sperm function, such as

watch out!

Prolonged treatment over more than a year to stimulate ovulation has been linked to a possible increase in the risk of ovarian cancer. Doctors don't know if this definitely occurs, but it is a possibility. You can discuss this with your specialist further if you are at all worried.

reduced ability of the sperm to move. As yet, no effective treatment has been proven to increase male fertility where the sperm function is impaired. This does not mean that nothing can be done. Effective treatment can be offered with the following assisted conception techniques:

• intracytoplasmic sperm injection (ICSI) (see pages 102–03), although there is a chance that conception may still occur naturally

• donor insemination (see pages 104–09). The decision to embark on this line of treatment requires careful consideration and counselling from specialist clinics.

Treating blocked fallopian tubes

One episode of pelvic infection can lead to infertility in up to 15 per cent of women. The more episodes of infection a woman has had, the greater the risk of tubal damage. It is therefore important that pelvic infection is treated promptly. Whether there has been pelvic infection, endometriosis or some other cause, sometimes the tubes are not actually blocked but are covered by adhesions at the ends or around the ovaries. These adhesions prevent release of the egg or stop the tube picking it up. In this instance, the best treatment is often in vitro fertilization (IVF) (see pages 94–7).

Alternatively, you could have tubal surgery to try to release the blockage, which is particularly useful if adhesions are stopping the release of the egg or preventing it from being picked up by the tube. While microsurgical techniques can be used to correct a mildly blocked tube, success rates are variable and not usually as effective as IVF.

must know

Risks from surgery
Surgery carries a ten per cent risk of a subsequent ectopic pregnancy. In addition, the greater the level of tubal damage, the lower the likelihood of successful surgery and subsequent pregnancy.

Reversing sterilization

Most women are happy with their decision to get sterilized. It is a highly effective method of contraception that is not designed to be reversible. But sometimes circumstances change and a couple want to try again for a baby. Sterilization is most commonly performed using keyhole or laparoscopic surgery. The tubes are blocked by a small plastic clip or ring that is surgically placed across them. Occasionally, sterilization is carried out by removing part or all of the tubes at the time of surgery. These procedures stop the sperm and egg from meeting.

Sterilization can be reversed successfully in many cases, providing there is not too much damage to the tubes and there is a reasonable

Sterilization with fallopian tubes blocked by clip.

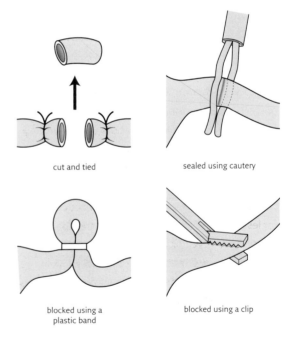

cut and tied

sealed using cautery

blocked using a
plastic band

blocked using a clip

amount of healthy tube remaining. Obviously, if the tubes have been removed, this will not be possible. A surgical operation is required to rejoin the tubes. This is a specialized field, but microsurgery by an expert tubal surgeon has a reasonable chance of success. There is a small risk of ectopic pregnancy (around four per cent) after tubal surgery to reverse a sterilization. If your tubes have been removed or the damage is too extensive, then IVF is usually the best option (see pages 94–7).

Treating unexplained infertility

Unexplained infertility is diagnosed after the other causes of infertility have been excluded. It accounts for about a quarter of all cases of infertility. If you have unexplained infertility and have been trying to get pregnant for less than three years, your chances of falling pregnant without treatment is as much as five to ten per cent per month. If you appear to have unexplained infertility and have been trying to get pregnant for more than three years, your chances of getting pregnant without treatment are around one to two per cent each month, so you will probably want to consider specialist treatment as soon as possible.

For younger women, a 'wait and see' policy can be adopted as some will conceive naturally, particularly if they have been trying to get pregnant for less than three years. Where you are older or the infertility has been present for more than three years, other options should be considered. The treatments are ovulation induction (see pages 81–2) or to use assisted conception techniques like IVF (see pages 94–7).

must know

Vasectomy reversal
Around ten per cent of men that have undergone vasectomy for sterilization subsequently want the procedure reversed, so that they can have more children, often with a new partner. Reversal is carried out surgically and microsurgical techniques appear best. Success will depend on the type of vasectomy performed and the length of time since the operation. The longer the time, the less chance of success. Indeed there is some evidence to suggest that success is most likely if reversal is carried out within five years of the vasectomy and success rates of over 90 per cent are achievable. After more than five to ten years have elapsed, success is less likely, but often still well over 50 per cent.

4 Assisted conception

Treatment of fertility problems have been revolutionized by assisted conception techniques, bringing hope to many couples who could not otherwise have had a baby. Assisted conception is the use of fertility treatments to bring sperm and egg together and so facilitate conception and pregnancy. The main techniques are in vitro fertilization (IVF), intracytoplasmic sperm injection (ICSI), intrauterine insemination (IUI) and donor insemination (DI).

Assisted conception clinics

There are now a large number of assisted conception clinics in the UK – over 80, in fact. Some of these clinics see only private patients and others see both private and NHS patients in the UK.

Where to go

A good starting point is to ask your GP about the clinics that are available in your area and whether they can provide a full range of fertility treatments. You will then want to know:

- what types of services the clinics offer
- what types of patients they see (private only or NHS and private?) It's not unusual for the same clinic to provide NHS and private treatment using the same facilities and laboratories
- if your GP is able to support any treatment you have, particularly if it is being carried out on a private basis, with the costs of drugs or tests
- the success rates of treatments at the clinics (see also below)
- the location of the clinics and if they have satellite centres (see also below)
- what their policy is on the number of embryos they transfer
- how often multiple pregnancies occur with each type of treatment
- if they have special features, such as sperm and egg donation programmes (see pages 104–09) or preimplantation genetic diagnosis (see pages 98–9)
- how long you will have to wait before being seen, and then how long it will take for your treatment to be carried out if you go ahead

did you know?

Clinic information

The website of the Human Fertilization and Embryology Authority (HFEA) (www.hfea.gov.uk) provides up-to-date information on all the clinics in the UK. It includes:
- The type of treatments they offer
- The numbers of each type of treatment they perform each year
- The success rates.

You can also contact clinics direct by telephone or website for more information.

• your elegibility for treatment. For example, some clinics only treat women under a certain age, even though there is no legal limit on the upper age limit. In addition, clinics can have different policies about treating same sex couples or single women

• if your treatment is being carried out privately, how much it would cost and what is and isn't included for that price. This can vary considerably from clinic to clinic (see pages 90–1).

Clinic success rates

Age is very important with regard to the success of fertility treatment (see graph, below) so when considering success rates, take into account the age of the women treated. The HFEA website (see details in box, opposite) shows the results for different treatments in various age groups, breaking it down into women below 35 years, those aged 35–37 years, those aged 38–39 years, and, those aged 40–42 years of age.

Graph illustrating the effect of the mother's age on fertility treatment success.

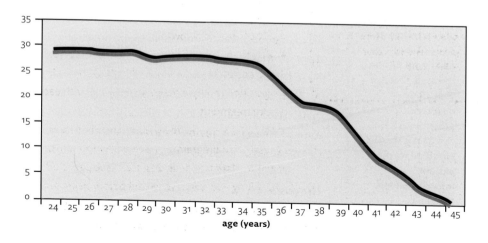

age (years)

Assisted conception success rates can also be gauged according to what part of the treatment process it is based on. For example, is the live birth rate based on the number of treatment cycles, the number of egg collections or the number of embryo transfers? The live birth rate is lower if it is based on cycles started rather than embryo transfers as not all treatment cycles lead to an egg collection. Sometimes the cycle has to be abandoned if the ovaries do not respond and too few or too many eggs develop.

In addition, not all eggs are fertilized successfully with a process like IVF and so treatment is also expressed as the number of live births for every embryo transferred back into the womb. Whether the embryo is fresh or frozen can also make a difference to the success rates with slightly lower success rates when the embryo has been frozen and stored.

Clinic location

Fertility treatment can be very stressful for both of you and it can be a time-consuming and emotional process that seems to take over your every waking thought. A clinic far from your home or workplace can add to the stress. Treatment involves frequent clinic attendances for the various procedures and by their very nature, they are not always carried out at the most convenient times. So travelling a long way to a clinic can add to the strain and make fertility treatment even more difficult to cope with.

To try to ease this, some clinics have so-called satellite units, based in local hospitals or clinics, which can carry out some of the tests or treatments without the need for you to visit the main centre for all components of your treatment.

The costs

There are different components to assisted conception treatment and costs are associated with each of them.

did you know?

Reducing costs

Egg sharing is a scheme operated by some clinics where, if you choose to donate some of the eggs collected from you following an IVF cycle to another woman who is unable to produce eggs, the price of your treatment can be reduced. Check if your clinic operates a scheme such as this as it is usually specified on the patient information for the clinic.

These include:

- the first clinic attendance and follow-up visits
- investigations, including hormone tests and sperm analysis
- ultrasound or X-ray examinations
- the cost of drugs, which can be very expensive
- blood tests and ultrasound examination to check on the egg development
- recovery of the eggs
- the fertilization procedure used, such as IVF
- the need for egg or sperm donation
- storage of embryos

This might add up to a significant total, but will vary from clinic to clinic. So if cost is a consideration, enquire whether there are any ways to reduce them.

The risk of twins

In the UK, fertility clinics only replace one or two embryos. Obviously, if two embryos both successfully implant, then you will have twins. You should, however, be aware that twin pregnancy carries a much higher risk of complications than a singleton pregnancy and because of this, some clinics are now performing only a single embryo transfer. Replacing only one embryo reduces the risk of a successful pregnancy compared to replacing two, but this is traded off against a lower risk of complications during a subsequent pregnancy. Your spare embryos can be frozen, stored and replaced at a later date.

Special features that clinics might provide

You may want to know if the clinic provides access to sperm donors or egg donors (see pages 104–09) or special services, such as preimplantation genetic diagnosis (see pages 98–9).

did you know?
Twin success rates in the UK

- For women under 35 years of age, the rate of twins in successful IVF pregnancies is 25–30 per cent.
- This declines to 18–19 per cent for women aged 38–39 years and even further for women over 40.

A clinic's assessment of your circumstances

In the UK, the Human Fertilization and Embryology Act, which was passed in 1990, requires clinics to consider the welfare of any baby that may be born by assisted conception therapy and the welfare of other children that might be affected by the birth of a new baby. So the clinic you opt for will have to ask you a number of personal questions to confirm your ability to meet the needs of a new baby as well as any medical factors that may be relevant. This may include the clinic contacting your GP to obtain relevant information from your medical records. However, before the clinic can do this, they must obtain consent from you.

Obtaining NHS treatment

There is some variation with regard to what treatment is offered on the NHS through different regions in the UK. However, in general, the NHS aims to offer women up to the age of 39 years at least one cycle of IVF without charge. Indeed, the National Institute for Clinical Excellence (NICE) recommends that IVF treatment should be offered to couples: in which the woman is aged between 23 and 39 years at the time of treatment; who have an identifiable cause for their fertility problems; and who have been infertile for at least three years. They should be offered up to three stimulated cycles of IVF. Despite these national guidelines, some criteria may be determined locally with regard to NHS treatment, such as whether or not one or other partner already has a child.

In addition, if, after investigation of your fertility problem, a specific cause is found that can be treated, the underlying condition would be treated rather than proceeding to assisted conception treatment. Assisted conception therapy would only be recommended if there is a reasonable chance of success. Usually your GP can advise you if you are eligible for NHS-funded assisted conception treatment.

Counselling

It is recommended that all couples with fertility problems are offered counselling by their clinic. This is because the diagnosis and treatment for fertility can be something that you and your partner find hard to deal with. It can cause problems with your relationship and so it is often good to talk it through with someone else who is removed from the situation.

Assisted conception clinics will offer you the opportunity of counselling to discuss the implications of the treatment you are planning on using. This ensures that you really understand what is involved in the process and how it will affect you, your partner and your family. A particularly important issue that you should talk through with your partner is using donated eggs or sperm. If this option applies to you, it is vital that you explore how both you and your partner feel about the related issues, as well as considering any legal implications before deciding if this is the right treatment for you.

Once you embark upon fertility treatment, you may require additional support and just one or two sessions with a counsellor can help you get through what can be a daunting and emotionally exhausting process. This kind of support can be particularly helpful if you have not managed to achieve a successful pregnancy.

did you know?

Counselling
Visiting a counsellor gives you the chance to talk easily about your emotions. It allows you to explore your feelings and gain support in finding the right path for you, by helping you to understand the issues involved, without feeling judged in any way.

About in vitro fertilization (IVF)

The phrase 'in vitro fertilization' means that the fertilization occurs 'in glass' in the laboratory. The eggs recovered after ovulation induction are mixed with sperm in the laboratory to produce a fertilized egg that develops into an embryo. The embryo is then replaced into the woman's womb.

must know

Cycle suppression side effects

Side effects may include hot flushes and night sweats as you are experiencing hormonal changes similar to the menopause. You might also experience vaginal dryness, headaches and a change in the size of your breasts. All these side effects are reversible on stopping the treatment.

How IVF works

Ideally, the doctor will want you to produce several eggs in a single cycle. The techniques used vary a little between clinics and specialists but, in general terms, the overall process remains the same.

First, your menstrual cycle is suppressed so that the doctors have greater control when it comes to stimulating the production of eggs. The usual way of suppressing your cycle is with either a long-acting injection given once per month or a nasal spray taken daily. These are usually started before a specific fertility treatment cycle.

The hormones that are injected are called gonadotrophins and they stimulate the body to trigger egg production (see pages 8–9). They are injected either into a muscle or under the skin depending on the preparation used. Many women, after being shown how to do this, are comfortable injecting themselves at home, so avoiding the need to attend clinics for injections.

The response of the ovaries to this stimulation is checked by ultrasound. The frequency of checks will depend partly on your response to treatment, but will usually occur around two to four times. (Some checks involve measuring hormone levels in the blood.) An ultrasound probe is inserted into the vagina and the doctor is then able to see each ovary and the eggs developing within.

Once the eggs have reached maturity after ten to twelve days, a further injection is used to finalize the maturation of the eggs. This injection must be given about 36 hours before the eggs are collected and so timing is critical. This form of ovulation induction often stimulates the production of several eggs, which can be very useful as, after fertilization, there may be several embryos resulting from one cycle of treatment. Any embryos not used in this 'fresh' cycle of IVF can be stored and used over several subsequent cycles without the need to go through ovulation induction again.

Collecting the eggs

When the eggs have reached maturity, they are retrieved. The woman is injected with a drug to make her drowsy or a general anaesthetic. The eggs are then collected by passing a needle through the

watch out!

An uncommon but serious complication for the mother from injecting gonadotrophins is called ovarian hyperstimulation syndrome. This occurs when the ovaries respond too vigorously to the stimulation, and dramatic changes in the body, including fluid retention and a risk of blood clots, occurs. These drugs, therefore, require careful monitoring when they are used.

must know
IVF success rates
Using fresh embryos, the average success rate, per cycle of treatment started is:
• Almost 30 per cent (in some clinics this figure is higher) in women under 35 years of age; 23-24 per cent for women aged 35-37 years; around 18 per cent for women aged 38-39 years; around 10 per cent for women aged 40-42 years.
• Where frozen embryos are used, success rates are usually slightly lower. For example, in women below 35 years of age, the average success rate is around 18 per cent.

vagina into the ovary. The needle is guided into position using an ultrasound scan with the ultrasound probe in the vagina, then the eggs are sucked down the needle and passed to the laboratory. After the eggs have been collected , it is usual to give the woman progesterone tablets or vaginal suppositories to ensure that the lining of the womb is fully prepared for the embryo to implant.

Fertilizing the eggs

In the laboratory, the collected eggs are mixed with your partner's, or donor's sperm, if this is being used. Your partner will have provided a fresh sample of sperm shortly before the eggs are collected. The sperm is prepared just as for intrauterine insemination (IUI) (see pages 100–01) and the eggs and sperm are mixed together in a laboratory dish. After around 20 hours, the eggs are checked to see if fertilization has occurred. Those that have been fertilized are left for another one to two days to allow the embryos to form.

Transferring the embryos

Finally, a few days after fertilization, one or two healthy embryos are replaced into the woman's womb. To do this, the doctor or nurse inserts a plastic device called a speculum into the vagina to separate the walls, so allowing them to see the cervix or neck of the womb. A fine tube like a thin straw is inserted through the neck of the womb and one or two embryos replaced through the tube. If there are other healthy embryos, these can be frozen and stored and used in subsequent treatment cycles without the need for ovulation induction.

In the UK, it is usual for only one or two embryos to be replaced. However, there are some circumstances where three embryos may be replaced. Typically, this is in women who are over 40 years, where a maximum of three embryos can be transferred at any one time. However, if the couple are using donor eggs, the maximum number of embryos that can be transferred is always two because the woman who is donating the egg is younger as egg donors are not accepted after age 35. As a result, the likelihood of a successful pregnancy from these eggs is higher.

When IVF is used

• to treat tubal blockage

• unexplained infertility

• where there are problems with sperm count

• where ovulation induction (see pages 81–2) and intrauterine insemination (see pages 100–01) have been unsuccessful

• for older women

did you know?
Moving frozen embryos
If you have frozen embryos in storage from previous IVF cycles, these can be transferred to another clinic so that you can have an embryo transfer and a further opportunity to become pregnant. Clinics can arrange to transfer embryos, but you are likely to have to pay for this service.

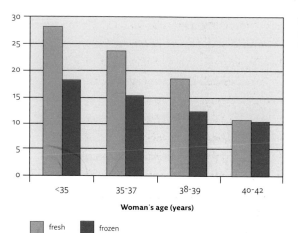

Typical success rates for IVF in the UK with fresh and 'frozen' embryo transfers.

fresh   frozen

Natural cycle IVF

This is an alternative procedure used where ovulation induction would not be suitable, such as for women who might be at high risk of thrombosis if ovulation induction is used, and where there is reliable egg production. The single egg produced each month is recovered and fertilized in the laboratory with your partner or donor sperm. Your doctor will advise you if this is a suitable treatment.

Testing for genetic disorders

Until recently, the only way to test if your unborn child had a genetic disease that may run in your family was to perform specific tests once the pregnancy was established and beyond twelve weeks' gestation. These tests carry a small but significant risk of causing a miscarriage (around one to two in every 100 tests) because they rely on taking the amniotic fluid from around the baby or some tissue from the placenta, using special needles under ultrasound guidance. These procedures can irritate the womb, leading it to contract, possibly resulting in miscarriage. Furthermore, if the fetus is found to have the genetic abnormality, all that can be offered is a termination of the pregnancy.

For couples with a known genetic abnormality, it is now possible to avoid these problems by using a technique in association with IVF called preimplantation genetic diagnosis (PGD). This is considered if you or your partner has a significant genetic disorder or if you have had another child with a genetic disorder. The disorders that can be picked up through PGD include haemophilia, an inborn bleeding tendency and cystic fibrosis, which can cause breathing and digestive problems. A small number of clinics offer this test and not all genetic disorders can be indentified in this way. If you do have a genetic disorder, your genetic counsellor can advise you.

How PGD works

With this type of treatment, the couple go through standard IVF. Then, once embryos are formed in the laboratory, they are tested to establish if any of them have the gene that causes the problem. The embryos are tested at a very early stage in their development when they are only tiny bundles of cells. A single cell is taken from each bundle and tested for the genetic disorder. Taking a cell from an embryo at this stage does not hinder the embryo's development in any way. In some cases, it may not be necessary to find the actual gene because just knowing the sex of the baby may be enough if a genetic disorder, such as haemophilia or Duchenne muscular dystrophy, only affects boys. In this situation, the sex of the embryo can be determined and only the female embryos will be replaced.

Preimplantation genetic screening

If a woman over 35 years old is having IVF, then this method can be used to test for chromosome disorders such as Down's syndrome. This involves checking that the number of chromosomes in the embryos produced by IVF is the right number before putting the embryo back. Your fertility specialist can advise you if this is available and whether it would be suitable for you. As with PGD, there are only a small number of clinics in the country who are able to carry out this technically demanding procedure.

Intrauterine insemination (IUI)

In intrauterine insemination (IUI) the doctor inserts sperm from your partner or a donor into the womb at the same time as your ovaries are releasing an egg. The aim of this procedure is to increase your chances of conception.

How IUI works

On the day that treatment is to take place, your partner is asked to produce a sample of semen. The sperm is washed in the laboratory to remove all the seminal fluid from around the sperm. The most healthy sperm can also be selected at this stage. Once this process is complete, the sperm are placed into a small tube to allow them to be inserted into the womb.

There are two ways IUI can be used:

• during a stimulated cycle in conjunction with ovulation induction as for IVF (see pages 94-7). The development of the eggs is monitored by ultrasound and when they are sufficiently mature after ten to twelve days, IUI is performed

• during an unstimulated cycle, when no fertility drugs are used. In this situation, the sperm is injected into the womb between Days 12 and 15 (when Day 1 is the first day of your period). A simple urine test can help confirm the time that you produce an egg

Inserting the sperm

To insert the sperm into the womb, the doctor or nurse inserts a simple plastic instrument called a speculum into the woman's vagina to help keep the walls apart. The doctor can then see the cervix, the neck or the womb. A soft flexible tube, like a long thin straw, is threaded through the cervix and into the womb and the prepared sperm are inserted.

The whole process takes only a few minutes and is rather like having a vaginal examination. It is usually relatively painless, although it may be a little uncomfortable. In addition, you may experience some cramping, period-like pains.

When IUI is used

• For unexplained infertility.

• If a man's sperm count is low or the sperm have low motility making it difficult for them to reach the egg naturally.

• When cervical mucous is hostile to the sperm (see page 72).

must know

IUI success rates
• The success depends upon the woman's age but, on average, a pregnancy occurs in around 15 per cent of couples with each cycle of treatment.
• It is therefore worth having several cycles of IUI treatment and usually doctors recommend three to six treatment cycles before proceeding to a different technique, such as IVF.

Other techniques

Techniques such as IUI and IVF can treat many fertility problems, but the main advance for male factor infertility is undoubtedly a technique called ICSI. Of course, there are some instances where even this might be unsuitable for a couple and donor sperm may be required (see pages 104–09). Furthermore, where there is a female factor that cannot be overcome by a technique such as IVF, surrogacy should be considered (see pages 110–11).

Intracytoplasmic sperm injection (ICSI)

ICSI is the direct injection of a single sperm into the fluid inside the egg cell, called cytoplasm. For the woman, the treatment is just like IVF, with the ovaries being stimulated to produce several eggs. In the laboratory, each of the eggs is injected with a single sperm to cause fertilization.

must know
ICSI success rates
Around 70 per cent of eggs injected with a sperm fertilize successfully and live birth rates are compatible with IVF (see pages 94–7).

When ICSI is used

• It is a high-tech procedure that has revolutionized the treatment of male factor infertility where the sperm count is very low or the sperm are abnormally shaped or can't move properly. Until ICSI was developed, success in the treatment of this type of infertility was very limited.
• Where IVF has been unsuccessful.
• Where there are no sperm in the man's ejaculate because of an obstruction to sperm getting to the penis. In this situation, the sperm are obtained directly from the testicle itself by a minor surgical procedure.

Health concerns

ICSI has been used in the treatment of infertility since the early 1990s and thousands of children have been born following this treatment. Studies so far have found that the children born from IVF and ICSI pregnancies are just as healthy and do just as well as children who are conceived naturally. One concern, however, is that where ICSI is used to treat male factor infertility, where there is a problem with sperm fertilizing the egg, boys born from these pregnancies may inherit this infertility trait. As most children born from ICSI pregnancies are not yet old enough to have children, there is no conclusive evidence.

Gamete intrafallopian transfer (GIFT)

When GIFT is used to treat a fertility problem, gametes – the collective word for the eggs and sperm – are collected just as they are for IVF (see pages 95–6). The healthy eggs are mixed with the sperm and, using keyhole surgery, they are placed into the fallopian tubes. With this procedure, the conception does not occur in the laboratory, but in your body, where it normally occurs when the sperm and egg meet.

If your own eggs and sperm are being used, GIFT can be carried out at clinics not necessarily licensed by the HFEA. However, if donor eggs and sperm are being used, the treatment would have to be carried out in an HFEA licensed clinic.

When GIFT is used

• For unexplained infertility. As the sperm and eggs are placed directly into the tubes, it can only be used where the tubes are known to be working normally with no blockage or damage
• for men with a low sperm count or where the sperm may not be able to 'swim' well and so might have difficulty in getting all the way from the vagina to the fallopian tube on their own. GIFT gets around this problem by putting the sperm and egg together.

**must know
GIFT success rates**
About 25 per cent of couples treated with GIFT become pregnant in each treatment cycle, although the success rate varies with factors such as the woman's age.

Donor sperm and eggs

Even though doctors and scientists have made massive advances with assisted conception technologies over the last few decades, there are still some situations where donor sperm or eggs will have to be used.

How sperm and egg donation works

For sperm insemination, it is important to ensure that the woman is ovulating and that her fallopian tubes are not damaged, nor are there any other medical problems. The clinic may want to perform some routine tests to check on all of this first. Also, other treatment options should have been considered, such as ICSI (see pages 102–03) if there is a problem such as a very low sperm count.

It is important that the insemination occurs around the same time as an egg is produced each month, so timing is important. Ovulation prediction kits that measure the level of a certain hormone in urine can be very useful for timing ovulation and treatment. For some women, it is better if the egg production is stimulated by medication prior to the insemination to increase the chance of a pregnancy occurring (see pages 81–2), but generally if you are ovulating regularly, around six cycles of donor insemination are used without ovulation stimulation treatment. Ovulation stimulation increases the risk of twins or triplets and so requires careful monitoring (see page 91).

must know
Frequency of sperm use
In the UK, a donor's sperm can be used to help up to ten families deal with a fertility problem. This, of course, means that your child could be genetically related to several other people. If a child conceived by donor sperm plans to marry, they can check with the HFEA to find out if they are genetically linked to their prospective partner.

Donor sperm is usually stored frozen in special sperm banks. At the woman's most fertile time, the sperm is defrosted and is then placed onto the cervix or inside the womb in the course of an examination.

How egg insemination works

The egg donor (who has to be under 35 years of age) is checked for any genetic disease or infection, such as HIV. She is also told about how ovulation induction and egg collection are performed and the risks attached to these procedures. After the eggs are collected from the egg donor, they are mixed with the father's sperm or a donor's sperm (if a sperm donor is being used too). Sometimes ICSI may be required to introduce the sperm directly to the egg (see pages 102–03). Just as with IVF, the embryos are then transferred into the womb (see pages 96–7).

When donor sperm and eggs are used

• When the male partner has a very low sperm count, donor insemination is a real alternative to ICSI (see page 102). So, if the woman has no fertility problem, then donor insemination may be a technique that you would want to consider as it avoids going through the ovulation induction and IVF processes (see pages 94–7), which are required for ICSI.

• If you have a high risk of passing on a genetic disorder (but see also embryo donation, page 109).

• For women in a same sex relationship or those who are single.

must know

Insemination success rates

Just as with IVF and other techniques, donor insemination success rates fall as the woman's age increases.

• For a woman under 35 years, the success rate from donor insemination is around 15 per cent for each treatment cycle.

• For women aged 40–42 years, this falls to around four per cent.

• If a woman has had a medical problem, which has resulted in the ovaries being removed. Previous cancer therapy may have made the ovaries fail.

• If a woman's ovaries have failed to develop or she has reached a very premature menopause.

• This treatment may also occasionally be of use when other fertility treatments have failed or if a woman has had recurrent miscarriages.

Deciding to use the treatment

In the UK, 1,500–2,000 babies are born every year using donated sperm or eggs or sometimes donated embryos. So, this is a fairly common fertility procedure, but it can, nevertheless, be a difficult decision to make.

Coming to terms with fertility problems is not always easy. Thinking about using donated sperm, eggs or even embryos is a major decision for both you and your partner. You will have to talk about it very carefully as a couple, making sure that you are conscious of each other's feelings and sensitivities.

When you make the decision to use donated sperm or eggs, it is not uncommon to experience a whole variety of emotional reactions. You may feel sad that you cannot have a baby with the sperm or eggs from the man or woman that you love. Sometimes, you may feel angry at the situation. You may experience a sense of loss, rather like a bereavement, when you discover that you cannot conceive, even with assisted conception, and that donated eggs or sperm will be needed. You may feel guilt or blame yourself when your eggs or sperm can't be used or feel that you have somehow let your partner down.

You may worry about what your partner is thinking or feeling.

It is not surprising, therefore, that when both of you are trying to come to terms with all of this, there can be some strain on your relationship, especially as each of you may cope in different ways with the emotions you are experiencing. This is a particular situation where counselling and support groups can be invaluable to help you make the right decision for you. Your fertility clinic will be able to help you identify local support groups and help you access counselling services that you may need. Take time to reflect on your decision and remember that a family is not just about passing on your own genes to your children, as thousands of families who have successfully had children using donated sperm or eggs can reassure you.

Choosing a sperm donor

When you decide to embark on this type of treatment, doctors at your fertility clinic will try to match the characteristics of the donor to you or your partner. Of course, this doesn't mean the baby will have definite similarities to you and your partner, but then neither does nature. Sometimes, if you are from a particular ethnic group, it may be difficult to obtain a close match to the characteristics that you want. In this situation, it is important to discuss all the options of finding the right donor with your doctor. However, you will not be able to identify the donor when selecting the characteristics that you wish for your child.

must know

Donor screening
Donors are carefully screened to exclude those with serious medical conditions and the donors are tested for infectious problems such as HIV and hepatitis.

It is possible to bring your own donor if there is someone who would be prepared to do this for you and if you would be comfortable with this type of arrangement. In this situation, the donor still has to go though the same screening for chronic viral infection like HIV, as any other sperm donor does. It takes at least six months for all the screening to be completed.

If you subsequently want to have another child using donor insemination, clinics generally try to ensure that the same sperm donor is available. So provided there is sufficient sperm available, and the donor has given consent, there should not be any problems.

Sperm donor anonymity

All people born through donor insemination can find out certain information through the HFEA once they are 18 years old. The information includes the donor's date and country of birth, their ethnic group, a physical description and recorded information about their medical history. Sometimes, the donor might provide more information, such as occupation and their reasons for donation. Donors may even leave a goodwill message for a child.

This information can be given by the HFEA without identifying the donor. When a donor has registered after April 2005, then the child conceived using the donor eggs or sperm, can apply to the HFEA to obtain identifying information about the person who gave the donation. This information includes their name, age and place of birth, their most recently known address and information about their physical appearance.

Because of this change in the legislations surrounding donations, you may want to consider how you would react if your child wants to learn more about or even contact the donor when they reach adulthood.

Choosing an egg donor

The fertility clinic is able to advise you on how best to identify a donor. They may have a waiting list for egg donors and, if so, they can give you some idea as to how long you might have to wait. It is also possible for you to ask relatives or friends if they would donate eggs for you. Sometimes you may even consider advertising for a suitable egg donor. A particular scheme that helps egg donation is called egg sharing. With egg sharing, a woman who is undergoing IVF treatment can donate some of her eggs to be used to treat another woman who is seeking an egg donor.

did you know?
The legal mother
The law in the UK states that it is the woman who is having the fertility treatment and the pregnancy who is legally considered to be the baby's mother and not the egg donor.

Embryo donation

Embryo donation might be something you would consider if both of you have significant fertility problems that cannot be easily treated using your own eggs and sperm. Sometimes it is of value when you do not want to pass on a genetic disease. Just as with sperm and egg donation, the clinic carrying this out for you would try to ensure that you had an embryo from donors who had physical characteristics similar to you. People who donate embryos have often themselves completed successfully a course, or several courses, of assisted conception treatment and they still have embryos available.

Surrogacy

Surrogacy is the situation where another woman carries the baby and gives birth to it for you. She is called the surrogate mother. It is usually the route chosen if the woman has a medical problem that means she cannot carry a pregnancy.

How surrogacy works

Depending on your condition, it may be that the embryo that the surrogate has implanted is created from your partner's sperm and your own eggs (known as partial surrogacy). In this instance, fertilization is carried out using IVF techniques (see pages 94–7).

Alternatively, the embryo is created from donated eggs from another woman and fertilized with your partner's sperm. This is known as full surrogacy. Usually the sperm is introduced by artificial insemination or intrauterine insemination (see pages 100–01).

Deciding to use surrogacy

Embarking on surrogacy is something that you should consider long and hard to ensure it is the right decision for you both. Surrogacy can have many difficulties so it is essential that both you and the surrogate are fully committed and you understand everything that is involved – not only the procedure, but what can happen in the years ahead. This is one situation where an experienced counsellor can be invaluable and help you make the right decision.

You and the surrogate have to trust each other and it is important to think through how you might feel about a surrogate carrying and delivering your baby. You also have to consider how you would deal with family and friends as well as any other children you or the surrogate may have. In the unfortunate and unlikely event that the baby is born with a serious congenital abnormality, you need to think how you would handle the situation.

Furthermore, the surrogate is the legal mother of the child and so her name is put on the birth certificate. This remains until the legal parentage of the baby is transferred through adoption or a parental order. The legal father of the child is usually the surrogate's partner and his name is put on the birth certificate.

Adoption is the procedure to follow if there is no genetic link between you and the baby. However, when the baby is genetically related to you and/or your partner, a parental order is used. When you apply for a parental order, both the surrogate and the father of the child must give their consent for this to be done and it has to be applied for within six months of the birth. Whatever route you choose, always take legal advice.

It is also important to understand that surrogacy can go wrong. The surrogate can change her mind about giving the baby to you at any point. Indeed, she can do this even if the baby is not genetically related to her. This is a very difficult emotional and painful situation for all concerned and emphasizes the need to ensure that there is a substantial degree of trust and commitment between you and the surrogate when you plan the pregnancy.

did you know?
Scottish law
In Scotland, it is possible for your partner to be named on the birth certificate so that he is the legal parent.

Finding a surrogate

In the UK, it is illegal for a clinic to find a surrogate for you, so you have to find her yourself. A good starting point is to talk to relatives or friends. Other people prefer to find a surrogate who is not related or known to them. It is illegal to advertise for a surrogate in the UK and you cannot pay a surrogate, although you can help with what is termed 'reasonable expenses' that the surrogate may incur as a result of carrying the baby for you.

5 You're pregnant!

Finding out you are pregnant is an exciting event. However, it is also often a time of increased anxiety. Very quickly you will notice your body changes as it adapts to meet the needs of your developing baby. But this transition is not just physical, it is also emotional and psychological. The pregnancy hormones affect how your brain functions, so that your emotions are heightened, with more extreme reactions to happy and sad events. This is all perfectly normal.

Finding out you're pregnant

You might suspect that you are pregnant even before you miss a period or take a pregnancy test. Many women become aware of changes in their body at a very early stage and are not that surprised to find out that they are pregnant.

Establishing pregnancy

The most common catalyst for taking a pregnancy test is missing your period. If you normally have a regular cycle and miss your period, you should always think about the possibility of pregnancy and perform a pregnancy test. Of course, missing a period doesn't always mean you are pregnant. Your menstrual cycle can be affected by stress, such as that due to a bereavement or to exam pressure, jet lag or sudden weight change. Never just assume that a factor like stress is the reason why your period is late. Even if you think pregnancy is not possible, for example, if you have been using the pill, then you should still think about pregnancy if you are having intercourse. Contraception might fail, for example, if you have an illness with vomiting and diarrhoea. If at all concerned about late or irregular periods, you should discuss this with your doctor.

Performing a pregnancy test
The easiest way to confirm your pregnancy is to purchase a pregnancy test kit – available from all pharmacies. Alternatively, you could visit your doctor, who will arrange to perform a pregnancy test for you.

Pregnancy tests measure a specific pregnancy hormone, secreted only by the placenta and known as human chorionic gonadotrophin (hCG). This hormone passes from the placenta into the bloodstream. It then passes through the kidneys and is detectable in urine in early pregnancy. Modern pregnancy tests are very reliable – more than 95 per cent accurate – and easy to use. The best results are to be had from urine obtained as soon as you get up in the morning, as it is in its most concentrated form at this time.

Some tests are more sensitive than others and are able to detect very low concentrations of hCG in the urine and may give a positive reading even before your period is missed. If it is negative, however, wait a few days; if your period has still not started, repeat the test.

Emotional changes

Many women find that they experience a mixture of emotions: a combination of the joy and excitement of pregnancy and, with your first baby, the anxiety you might feel about the changes in your lifestyle and the increased responsibility that a baby brings. You might also feel anxious about the possibility of complications during pregnancy. It often helps to share your feelings with your partner, relatives and friends. Talk to other mothers-to-be; you will probably find that despite their confident, happy exterior, inside they have the same whirl of emotions and worries as you.

must know

Doing a pregnancy test

The precise instructions vary from brand to brand (always read and follow the manufacturer's instructions), but all work on the same principle.
• Collect some of your urine and drop it onto the test stick or hold the stick under your stream of urine.
• Wait for about five minutes to see the result.
• If positive, the result may be displayed in the 'window' of the test stick as two blue lines or as a red cross or two pink dots. Sometimes your doctor will measure the pregnancy hormone hCG in your blood to confirm that you are pregnant.

Morning sickness

About half of all pregnant women experience morning sickness. Nausea and morning sickness usually start a few weeks after conception, although some lucky women do not suffer from these at all throughout their entire pregnancy.

did you know?

The baby's health

Your baby isn't harmed by morning sickness. Indeed, it is thought to be a sign of a well-established pregnancy. It can lead you to lose weight in early pregnancy, but don't worry about the baby, his or her growth will not be affected. Your baby gets all the nourishment it needs from your body stores.

What is morning sickness?

Morning sickness is a misleading name as, although it is common in the morning, it can occur at any time of day. It may be worse when your stomach is empty, hence the association with the morning. It can also be worse when you are tired. It isn't known precisely what causes morning sickness, but it is probably related to the hormonal changes in your body due to the implanting pregnancy. It is usually most severe when the levels of hCG are highest in the first three months of pregnancy and the sickness tends to resolve as levels decline in the second three months. However, for a small number of women, it can persist for much longer. In fact, occasionally some women can experience it throughout the pregnancy.

If you are not coping very well, keep a record of how much food and fluid you are managing to keep down and get help from your doctor. Severe morning sickness can lead to dehydration that can make you ill, so drinking plenty of water every day is important. But do still try and take your folic acid vitamin supplements, even if you feel sick; you may have to adjust the time you take your tablets. If you are on iron tablets to prevent anaemia, these may aggravate the condition and need to be withheld until the morning sickness settles.

Do not take any medication to combat morning sickness unless prescribed by your GP. For severe cases there are medicines that help to control the sickness, but you must consult your GP, who can give you specific tailored advice for your own situation.

Hyperemesis gravidarum

Hyperemesis gravidarum is the medical name for a very severe form of morning sickness:
- 'hyper' = a large amount of
- 'emesis' = sickness
- 'gravidarum' = in pregnancy

must know

Minimizing morning sickness
- Avoid any foods that make it worse.
- Take frequent small snacks so your stomach is not empty. Dry biscuits or dry toast are good, especially in the morning. Keep some biscuits by the bed so you can eat something before you get out of bed.
- Some women find that acupressure on a point on the wrist (known as the 'neiguan point') relieves nausea. Wrist bands used for travel sickness put pressure on this point and may be worth trying, too.

The condition is uncommon, occurring in less than one per cent of pregnancies. It usually starts between six and eight weeks after your last menstrual period and tends to continue until about 20 weeks. Occasionally it can last throughout the pregnancy.

Morning sickness becomes hyperemesis when you have persistent nausea with vomiting several times a day, leading to dehydration, with biochemical upset in your body and inadequate nutrition, leading to weight loss. Unfortunately, it tends to recur in subsequent pregnancies, so if you have had it once, you are likely to have it again. Sometimes there is also a mild upset of liver function.

Doctors don't yet know why hyperemesis occurs. However, it is known that there is a link with high levels of hCG. This may be why hyperemesis is more common in twin pregnancies as, with two placentas, the level of hCG is much higher. High levels of hCG in your blood can cause the thyroid gland to become slightly overactive on a temporary basis, which might partially account for all the nausea and vomiting. Another possible cause is stomach infection with the bacterium Helicobacter pylori, known to cause stomach ulcers. A psychological component to hyperemesis has also been proposed.

If you have severe morning sickness or think that you may have hyperemesis gravidarum, seek advice from your doctor or midwife. There are many ways that your doctor or midwife can help you. These range from simple measures to do with diet or eating pattern, to specific medication. It is important to get treatment before you are at risk of complications. Dehydration, vitamin deficiencies or blood clots can occur if the sickness continues unchecked.

Treating hyperemesis gravidarum

Women with hyperemesis gravidarum are usually admitted to hospital. Treatment includes fluids given through a vein to rehydrate the mother, medication to reduce the nausea and vomiting, and vitamin supplements to replace lost nutrients. Steroid medication can be effective in severe cases. Occasionally, intravenous feeding is required and medication can also be given to reduce the risk of blood clots.

Despite such complications being dangerous for the mother, there is no evidence of an increased risk of abnormality in the developing baby. However, in particularly severe cases, where a woman loses more than 5 per cent of her body weight, there is a higher chance of the baby being small.

must know

Changing palette
It is very common to go off certain foods and drinks during pregnancy. You may find that you don't like the taste of alcohol or can't drink coffee. Many women describe a metallic taste in their mouth. Your sense of smell may also become more sensitive, so that the smell or taste of certain foods can make you feel nauseous. It is not known why this happens, but it may be nature's way of protecting the baby from potentially harmful substances, like alcohol, at a critical stage in the baby's development.

Your changing body

Once you conceive, you will notice many changes in your body, some will occur quickly and others will occur more gradually. Some of the changes can sometimes be alarming so it is important to know how your body might react to the pregnancy establishing itself.

Your breasts

One of the most noticeable early changes in your body happen to your breasts.

• They may get bigger even before you miss your period. You will probably notice that your bra is beginning to feel a bit tight.

• They may also feel tender and you may have a tingling sensation. Or they may feel lumpy to touch and seem extremely itchy.

• The veins on your breasts can become very obvious too, especially if you have pale skin. This is because of an increase in blood supply to prepare them for breastfeeding.

• Your nipples also enlarge and become darker in colour, as well as being very sensitive to touch. The pigmented skin round each nipple, called the areola, develops small raised glands known as Montgomery's tubercles, which produce an oily secretion that lubricates and protects the skin of the nipples during breastfeeding.

It is important to wear a bra that fits properly to minimize the discomfort. Remember that breast size changes throughout pregnancy and you may need to be re-measured.

Tiredness

Many women feel very tired in the early stages of pregnancy. It is not unusual to feel that you have to sleep in the afternoon or early evening, even when you would not normally do so. The reason you feel tired is because your body is adapting to meet the demands of your developing baby. If you are worried about tiredness or it continues or is severe, consult your doctor. Occasionally, tiredness can be due to anaemia, which can be checked by a blood test and is easily treated by iron and vitamin supplements (see page 32).

Passing urine frequently

When you are pregnant, it is common to need to pass urine more often because of the pressure of the enlarging womb (uterus) on your bladder. Although urinary frequency is normal, pain on passing urine is not and could indicate a bladder infection (cystitis), which should be treated promptly, especially in pregnancy. You must see your GP at once.

Vaginal discharge

Secretions from your vagina increase in pregnancy. This is due to the increase in blood flow in your pelvis. The discharge is normally clear or white in colour. If it is yellow, green or bloodstained, smells offensive or is accompanied by itching, discomfort or ulceration, then you must tell your doctor. A bloodstained discharge may indicate a threatened miscarriage, for instance (see pages 154–62).

did you know?
Thrush
An abnormal discharge in pregnancy is most commonly due to a yeast infection called thrush (candida infection). It causes itching and irritation round the vulva and vagina and often has a thick white or yellow discharge that can be described as 'curd-like'. It is easily treated by a course of pessaries or creams. The infection is confined to the skin alone and does not affect the baby or harm the pregnancy in any way.

Skin changes

As well as darkening of the nipples, other pigment changes occur in your body in pregnancy. This is because high levels of oestrogen (the female hormone produced in increased quantities when you are pregnant) increases the ability of your skin to produce pigment. These changes are normal. The thin line that appears in pregnancy running from your pubic area to the navel (umbilicus) is called the 'linea nigra'.

If you have freckles, these often darken in pregnancy, too. You may also notice that any recent scars and even your genital area become more pigmented. In darker-skinned people, pigmented vertical lines can appear on the fingernails in pregnancy. You also find that you tan more readily, although it may be more patchy than usual.

Patchy pigmentation can also occur on the face around the chin, forehead, nose and mouth; this is known as chloasma, the so-called 'mask' of pregnancy. It probably affects about half of all pregnant women to a greater or lesser degree and is more common in brunettes than in blondes. It can also occur in women taking the combined (oestrogen-containing) contraceptive pill.

To help reduce pigmentation, use a high-protection sunscreen when exposed to the sun. Any changes can usually be camouflaged with cover-up cosmetics. If the changes are marked and cause you concern, seek specialist medical advice. Once the baby is born, they fade and the skin usually returns to normal.

Other changes to the skin, such as palms looking redder and the appearance of little red 'spider-like' blood vessels, are also due to the high oestrogen levels and an increased blood flow to the skin. Over ten per cent of white women have vascular 'spiders' by the second month of pregnancy and two-thirds have them by term. They are less common in black women, affecting fewer than 15 per cent by term. Over half of all women develop red palms in pregnancy, which is known as 'palmer erythema'.

Bleeding gums and dental decay

Changes in your gums are probably related to the hormonal changes of pregnancy. Some softening of the gums, together with increased blood supply, can make your gums more likely to bleed after brushing as well as more prone to gingivitis (inflammation of the gums). Such changes are common in pregnancy, affecting around a third of pregnant women, and can appear early on.

Dental decay can also worsen in pregnancy. It is important, therefore, to brush and floss your teeth regularly, and it is usually advisable to see your dentist at least once during pregnancy.

did you know?
Greasy skin
The changes in your hormones in pregnancy often lead to more oil production by the skin. Regular use of a clarifying lotion on your face can help, along with a moisturising cream that is designed for oily skin. If you use make-up, find one with an oil-free base. If you find you get troublesome acne or spots, consult your GP. Do not take any medication for acne without discussing it with your doctor first as some preparations might potentially harm the baby.

Estimated date of delivery

Almost as soon as you are pregnant you will want to know when to expect your new arrival. This is not just for the wonder and excitement of seeing this new life that you have created, but also for practical reasons; to plan and organize the nursery, maternity and paternity leave and to buy those first baby clothes.

must know

Ultrasound and delivery dates

• It is critical to have a good assessment of the stage of your pregnancy in case complications arise. It is best, therefore, to confirm your dates by an ultrasound scan.

• Convention has always related gestation to the first day of the last menstrual period, so for women who know the date of conception, such as those undergoing assisted conception, the duration of pregnancy from conception is 38 weeks rather than 40.

• While every woman is given an EDD, very few women will deliver on that day. It is normal for you to go into labour at any time between 37 and 42 weeks.

Calculating when your baby is due

The estimated date of delivery (EDD) is calculated as 40 weeks (280 days) from the start of your last menstrual period. Conception usually occurs two weeks after the last period and the duration of the pregnancy is 38 weeks (266 days) from conception. But this only applies if:

• you have a regular four-week cycle

• the first day of the last period is certain

• there has been no bleeding since your last period

• no contraception was being used (if you conceived after coming off the pill then the last menstrual period is not reliable for calculating your dates)

So while your doctor will use your last period to calculate a provisional EDD, this is usually checked against the result of an ultrasound scan.

A long or short menstrual cycle

If you have a menstrual cycle that is longer than 28 days – say, 35 days – but regular, then the estimated date of delivery can be calculated by adding 41 weeks to the first day of your last period. Conversely, if you have a regular 21-day cycle, the estimated date of delivery is calculated by adding 39 weeks to the last day of the menstrual cycle. If you have an irregular cycle or a cycle that is longer than 35 days, the EDD cannot be estimated reliably from the starting date of your last period.

did you know?

Calculating EDD
Nowadays, most Doctors and midwives use calculators to work out the EDD, but the rule is still useful and works fairly well with a regular 28-day cycle to give an estimate of the EDD.

Naegele's formula

This is a formula that doctors use as a quick way to calculate when a baby is due. It is based on the date of the last menstrual period. It only works when the start date of the woman's last menstrual period is known, where there is a regular 28-day cycle, and where no contraception was being used prior to conception.

How the formula is calculated

- add seven days to the starting date of your last menstrual period
- subtract 3 from the month
- add 1 to the year

Here is an example:
Your last menstrual period began on 8 May 2007 (8.5.2007)
- add 7 days to the day: $7 + 8 = 15$
- subtract 3 from the month (May being the fifth month): $5 - 3 = 2$ (February)
- add 1 to the year: $2007 + 1 = 2008$
- so the estimated date of delivery is: 15 February 2008

Your developing baby

Having an ultrasound scan is the final confirmation of the presence of a viable pregnancy in the womb and is usually carried out at your first visit to the obstetrician, usually by six weeks after the missed period.

must know

Measuring time
In pregnancy, weeks are measured from the start of your last menstrual period, although fertilization occurs about 14 days later.

Ultrasound scans

Most women feel very reassured by seeing their developing baby on the scan. It may be performed by the obstetrician or by a radiologist (a medical specialist in imaging), an ultrasonographer (a specialist ultrasound technician) or a midwife. The scan is usually carried out through the abdomen but the pregnancy may be detected slightly earlier if the scan is carried out through the vagina.

Before twelve weeks it is not possible to identify clearly the sex of your developing baby. There is a swelling in the genital region but it is only after twelve weeks that this forms a penis in a boy. Doctors usually wait until around 16–18 weeks, when the baby is bigger, before trying to determine the sex using an ultrasound scan.

Abnormalities

It is very unusual to see abnormalities on the first scan if this is carried out early in pregnancy, at six to twelve weeks. Ultrasound at this stage confirms that the baby is alive by showing the heartbeat and helps to assess the stage of the pregnancy by measuring the size of the developing fetus. Where scans are being performed to exclude abnormality in the baby, they are usually carried out later in pregnancy, at 16–20 weeks, when the baby has developed further and is large enough for the organs to show up adequately. A scan at this stage assesses very carefully the anatomy of the baby.

The developing baby in early pregnancy

The age of the embryo is assessed from six to twelve weeks by measuring the crown-rump length (the length from the top of the head to the bottom of the embryo). Thereafter, ultrasound is used, measuring the diameter of the head.

Age	Details
4 weeks	The gestation sac (the bag of fluid in which the baby grows) is approximately 3 mm ($^1/_{10}$ in) in diameter and the embryo just visible to the naked eye.
6 weeks	The gestation sac is around 2 cm ($^3/_4$ in) in diameter and the umbilical cord is formed. The embryo is less than 10 mm ($^1/_2$ in) long and a head and tail end are present. Ultrasound can show the fetal heartbeat.
8 weeks	The gestational sac is 3–5 cm ($^1/_4$–2 in) in diameter and the embryo is approximately 18 mm ($^2/_3$ in) in length. The limbs are well formed and toes and fingers are present.
10 weeks	The fetus is over 3 cm ($^1/_4$ in) long. The head is taking on a more recognizably human shape. The internal organs are formed and the limbs are becoming well defined.
12 weeks	The gestational sac is 10 cm (4 in) in diameter and the foetus is approximately 60 mm ($2^1/_2$ in) long. The skull bones can be seen clearly on a scan. The face has formed and finger- and toenails are starting to develop.

must know

Embryo vs fetus
The developing baby is known as an embryo until the eighth week of pregnancy. By then, the outward appearance of the fetus is recognizably human and from this stage until delivery it is known as a fetus.

The placenta

The placenta is essential as it acts as the interface between fetus and mother. A disc-shaped organ, it consists of a rich network of blood vessels derived from the fetus that implants into the wall of your womb very early in pregnancy. The placenta is linked to the fetus by the umbilical cord and is therefore the means by which the fetus is physically attached to the mother.

The placenta 'invades' the mother's blood vessels and so becomes bathed in the mother's blood, from which it is able to extract oxygen and nutrients. These are then transported to the fetus through its bloodstream. The blood going from the fetus to the placenta contains the carbon dioxide and waste products produced by the fetus. These are transferred to the mother's blood and the mother then excretes these for the fetus through her lungs and kidneys.

The placenta and umbilical cord.

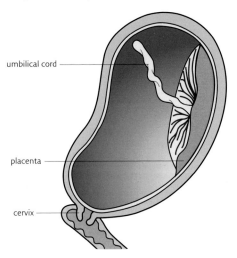

umbilical cord

placenta

cervix

The umbilical cord

This 'lifeline' connects the fetus to the placenta. It contains three major blood vessels: two umbilical arteries, which carry blood and waste products from the fetus to the placenta, and one umbilical vein, which carries blood, rich in oxygen and nutrients, from the placenta to the fetus. These vessels are encased in a jelly-like substance (the medical term is 'Wharton's jelly') which, in turn, is covered in a tough outer coating. The umbilical cord is often coiled so that there is plenty of 'give' to allow for fetal movement in the womb.

The amniotic fluid

In early pregnancy, the amniotic fluid comes from the membranes encasing the fetus and placenta. In late pregnancy the fluid is actually produced by the developing baby's kidneys and excreted as 'urine' (waste products still pass through the placenta to the mother who filters them out through her kidneys). Well-nourished babies produce lots of urine so there is plenty of amniotic fluid. This helps cushion the baby from any injury and allows it to move within the womb until 32 weeks or so when the size of the baby makes it difficult for the baby to move around. In a baby who is not receiving a good supply of nutrients, usually because the placenta is not working as well as it should, the amount of fluid is low. Marked reductions in amniotic fluid, usually assessed by ultrasound, are an important indication that the baby may have a problem.

Antenatal visits

The vast majority of women remain healthy during pregnancy – it's a natural state, after all, and not an illness. However, you can not take good health in pregnancy for granted. So, the purpose of antenatal care is to identify potential problems early on and treat them before they develop into a more severe complication.

The importance of regular checks

Serious problems can arise during pregnancy both for you and the baby. These problems might not only affect the pregnancy but can also affect you and your baby's future health. This is why regular checks by doctors and midwives during pregnancy are considered so important, indeed essential.

The aims of antenatal care

• To establish the stage of the pregnancy and your estimated date of delivery (EDD) in order to plan your care.
• To treat minor problems you might encounter in pregnancy, such as heartburn.
• To identify and treat any pre-existing medical conditions you may have, such as diabetes, epilepsy or heart disease.
• To check whether or not you are at risk of complications arising in pregnancy and, if possible, prevent these complications. For example, if you are at risk of anaemia, this can be prevented with iron and vitamin supplements.
• To offer screening for abnormalities in the fetus.
• To identify and treat any new problems you may develop in your pregnancy, such as pre-eclampsia (see pages 162–3).

- To make a plan for your labour and delivery.
- To provide information on infant feeding and care.
- To offer family planning advice, if required, for after delivery.
- To provide advice, reassurance, education and support for you and your family regarding all aspects of pregnancy, including postnatal exercises, baby care and issues relevant to your general health, such as smoking.

Healthcare professionals

Many healthcare professionals are involved in antenatal care. The main providers are GPs, midwives and obstetricians, but physiotherapists, dietitians and other professionals allied to medicine may be involved, depending on your needs. Antenatal care may be set in local community clinics or in hospital clinics or shared between community and hospital.

Care is organized to meet your particular needs. For example, if you have a medical problem like diabetes, you are usually seen at a specialist clinic. If you have no problems and have previously had one or more uncomplicated pregnancies and deliveries, then you are considered to be at low risk of developing complications and are therefore likely to receive most of your care in the community. Obviously, should a problem arise requiring more medical or 'high tech' input, this is provided. The important issue is to ensure you get the right level of care to meet your needs at every stage in your pregnancy.

The first visit

Once your pregnancy has been confirmed by your GP, you are referred to a hospital or community clinic for a first visit. This is usually eight to twelve weeks after your

did you know?

Make a list
A good tip is to make a list of all the things that you want to know or are concerned or anxious about. Before you leave the consultation, check that everything has been answered.

last period. Some women with particular pregnancy problems, such as heart disease or those on specific medication, such as anticoagulants for thrombosis, may need to be seen earlier, which is best planned pre-pregnancy. The earlier you confirm your pregnancy and attend your GP, the earlier you are seen at the clinic.

This first visit is usually the longest as you are asked detailed questions about various matters (see box, opposite). The information you provide determines if you are at risk of any particular problems in pregnancy and helps to identify the right pattern of antenatal care for your particular needs. In addition, screening for fetal abnormality is discussed (see pages 142–7), so you may want to think about how you feel having these tests before you attend the visit. You are also examined physically (see also box, opposite) .

Many women find that having their partner with them helps, not only as support, but also to remind them of the important questions they were thinking about before the visit and otherwise might have forgotten to ask. Never hesitate in asking questions if something is bothering you, no matter how trivial you think it may be.

If you have particular preferences about the type of care you want or how you want to deliver your baby, then raise these at your first visit. For many women, pregnancy – especially the first pregnancy or where a previous pregnancy has been complicated – can be a frightening experience, so it is essential that you and your partner raise all your anxieties and questions and discuss issues fully with the obstetrician or midwife.

What happens at the first visit to the antenatal clinic

The doctor or midwife asks for:
- details of your medical and family history
- details of any medication that you are on
- information on smoking, alcohol and drug use
- a detailed pregnancy history for any previous pregnancies
- the date of your last menstrual period and details about your menstrual cycle
- details of any contraception used and your last cervical smear test

Physical examination by the doctor includes
- taking your blood pressure (see page 138)
- an external examination of your abdomen – an internal (vaginal) examination is not usually required
- measuring your height and weight

Tests performed:
- urine check for infection and the presence of sugar and protein (see pages 136–7)
- blood tests to determine your blood group and to check for certain blood disorders (see pages 138–40)
- an ultrasound scan to confirm the stage of your pregnancy and to check for twins
- a cervical smear test, if you are due one, can be carried out safely

Future tests discussed:
- screening for fetal abnormality, such as nuchal ultrasound scan, triple test and detailed anomaly ultrasound scan (see pages 144–5)
- amniocentesis and chorionic villous sampling (CVS), if required (see pages 146–7)

must know

Urine specimens
It is very important to bring a urine specimen to every antenatal check. Checking the urine for protein is key to detecting women who are developing pre-eclampsia, a disorder associated with high blood pressure and which can be dangerous for both mother and baby. If you forget to bring a specimen you should try and produce one before you leave the clinic.

Subsequent antenatal visits

You are seen around every four weeks from diagnosis of pregnancy until week 28 of gestation, fortnightly until week 36 of gestation and then weekly until delivery. It is questionable whether low-risk woman with an uncomplicated pregnancy (see box, opposite) need so many assessments, but the correct frequency of assessment is not scientifically established and so this depends on the judgement of your doctor or midwife and should, of course, take into account your specific needs.

An assessment of your level of risk determines the type of care you require. This risk assessment is based on the medical information obtained at the first visit, the results of tests and any new complications or problems that develop. It is important to remember that your level of risk can rise and fall, as problems develop or resolve.

Examples of risk factors are shown in the box opposite. If you have no risk factors, you are designated 'low risk', but remember that risk factors such as pre-eclampsia and breech presentation can be 'acquired' later in pregnancy and will only be identified through good antenatal care and regular checks.

What happens at subsequent antenatal checks

The doctor or midwife ask you if:
• there have been any new problems
• you have been feeling your baby move (a sign of wellbeing)

Physical examination by the doctor includes:
• taking blood pressure (see page 138)
• an external examination of your abdomen to assess the size of your womb to ensure your pregnancy is growing normally
• checking how the baby is lying in the womb (in later pregnancy) and identifying whether or not the baby's head or bottom (breech) is in your pelvis

Tests performed:
• urine check for infection and the presence of sugar and protein (see pages 136-7)
• if you are rhesus negative (see pages 139-40), additional blood tests may be taken for anaemia and for rhesus antibodies

To assess the size of your womb, many doctors or midwives use a measuring tape. They measure from the pubic bone in the midline to the highest part of the womb, known as the fundus. The highest part is usually to one side of the midline, most commonly the right side as the womb often deviates to that side when it grows in pregnancy.

Risk factors for pregnancy and delivery

General risk factors
- age if under 20 and particularly under 16 or over 35 years
- the mother being very overweight or underweight
- more than four previous pregnancies
- pre-existing medical conditions, such as diabetes, blood clots or high blood pressure
- a history of alcohol or drug abuse
- a family history of fetal abnormality, genetic or chromosomal abnormality or problems with thrombosis

Past pregnancy problems
- previous Caesarean section(s)
- previous severe high blood pressure or pre-eclampsia
- previous pregnancy complicated by premature labour
- previous pregnancy complicated by an abnormality in the baby
- a small baby in a previous pregnancy (less than 2.5 kg (5 lb 8 oz) at birth)
- a very big baby in a previous pregnancy (more than 4.5 kg (10 lb) at birth)
- severe difficulty with delivery of the baby's shoulders in a previous pregnancy
- previous stillbirth or neonatal death
- recurrent miscarriages

Problems in the present pregnancy
- excess or reduced fluid around the baby
- threatened premature labour
- pre-eclampsia or high blood pressure
- twins or triplets
- a very big baby
- a very small baby
- breech presentation
- bleeding in pregnancy

Antenatal tests

When you go to your first antenatal visit, you will receive a lot of information. In addition, many tests and checks are carried out and it is often difficult to remember what all these are for, and why they are so important.

Urine checks

A urine sample is needed to check for the presence of protein and glucose (sugar), which are easily diagnosed on 'dipstick' testing of your urine.

• Protein in the urine can indicate a kidney problem, bladder infection or pre-eclampsia (see pages 162–3). Small amounts of protein can be found in the urine, however, if you have a bladder infection or if a bit of vaginal discharge gets into the urine specimen.

• Glucose can be found in your urine if there is a diabetes problem (see pages 166–8), but it is not uncommon for small amounts of glucose to be present in the urine in a normal pregnancy, especially if you have eaten something before producing the sample.

The urine is usually checked specifically for infection at your first visit, as bladder and kidney infections are more common in pregnancy and may be more severe.

Urinary tract infection

Urinary tract infection (UTI) is more common when you are pregnant and it is routine to check for a UTI at your first visit. The flow of urine through the tubes that lead from your kidneys to your bladder is slower during pregnancy due to the effects of the pregnancy hormone progesterone so making you more prone to infection.

Most commonly any pain passing urine is likely to be a simple bladder infection (cystitis). You will feel the need to pass urine frequently, it will be painful when you pass urine – usually a burning feeling – and you will feel a sense of urgency when you need to go to the toilet. Sometimes these infections can even lead to blood appearing in your urine. If the infection spreads from your bladder to your kidneys, you will feel very unwell. This is called pyelonephritis but it is not a common problem in pregnancy. If it occurs, you will have a fever, shiver and usually have loin pain and tenderness. It is not uncommon to feel nauseated and vomit.

Severe untreated infections can irritate the womb and lead to premature labour, so prompt treatment is necessary to stop the infection worsening to a stage that it can upset the pregnancy. Treatment is usually by a broad-spectrum antibiotic (an antibiotic that kills all the usual bacteria that cause UTIs). Most antibiotics are safe in pregnancy.

If you get repeated UTIs when you are pregnant, long-term antibiotic treatment may be given, usually at night, when the antibiotic stays in the bladder for several hours. With a UTI, drink plenty of fluids to ensure a good flow of urine to help flush the infection out of your bladder. Drinking cranberry juice is known to be helpful in fighting bladder infections.

Blood pressure checks

Blood pressure is measured so that the doctor or midwife can hear the systolic pressure – the highest point of your blood pressure – and the diastolic pressure – the lowest point of the blood pressure. When your blood pressure is recorded, the doctor writes, for example, 115/75. This means that your systolic pressure is 115 mmHg and your diastolic pressure is 75 mmHg.

High blood pressure is associated with an increased risk of having pre-eclampsia (see pages 162–3) and a small-for-dates baby (one that has not grown as big as it should have for the stage it has reached in pregnancy). You will require a little more antenatal care. However, the majority of women with high blood pressure will experience a successful pregnancy.

Blood tests

Several blood tests are taken at the first visit. These check for anaemia, identify your blood group, and see if you are immune to rubella. Syphilis is screened for as this sexually transmitted disease can affect the baby. Although infection during pregnancy is rare in the UK, it can be easily and safely treated to prevent the baby being born with a form of syphilis. Other infections like hepatitis are also screened for.

If there is a risk of certain blood disorders, such as sickle-cell anaemia (see pages 178–81), your blood is screened specifically for these. Some hospitals offer screening to determine if you and your partner are carriers of cystic fibrosis (a genetic disorder that causes chronic lung disease) and digestion difficulties. Additional blood tests are required if you have a particular medical disorder, such as blood-clotting problems, diabetes, heart disease or thyroid disease. HIV testing may be performed after counselling.

Blood groups and rhesus disease

Everyone has a blood group. Blood group typing comprises two main categories: ABO, consisting of groups A, B, AB or O; and rhesus, consisting of rhesus positive and rhesus negative. You are likely to see your blood group written in your pregnancy record: for example, it might be 'A Rh+', meaning that you are blood group A and rhesus positive. 85 per cent of people are rhesus positive and 15 per cent rhesus negative.

A problem can sometimes arise if you are rhesus negative and you are carrying a rhesus positive baby. Some of the baby's blood cells can leak into your bloodstream during the pregnancy. The risk of the baby's cells entering your bloodstream is higher when bleeding occurs in pregnancy. Because you are rhesus negative, your body recognizes that these rhesus positive cells are not yours. It regards them as foreign cells and responds by making antibodies (substances that attack and destroy foreign cells – in the case of infection, for example). The antibodies that you produce against rhesus positive cells can cross the placenta and enter your baby's bloodstream. If levels of the antibodies are high, they can cause the developing baby to become anaemic by destroying the red blood cells in the baby's bloodstream, which will all be rhesus positive. This is called rhesus disease.

must know

Safety precautions
Following delivery, a mother's blood is checked with the Kliehauer test to determine how much of the baby's blood has entered her bloodstream. This is done to ensure she has had enough anti-D immunoglobulin to clear all of the baby's red cells. This can prevent repetition of the problem in her next pregnancy if the baby is rhesus positive again.

However, this is becoming less and less common in the UK because, soon after any bleeding in pregnancy and after delivery, rhesus negative mothers are injected with an antibody called anti-D immunoglobulin (many hospitals also give it routinely at around 28 and at 34–36 weeks during the pregnancy). The injections help clear the baby's red blood cells from the mother's bloodstream, preventing her from making these antibodies and so preventing rhesus disease.

If mother and baby are rhesus negative, this problem cannot occur. The baby's blood group is not known, however, until after delivery when the blood group will be checked or some blood taken from the umbilical cord.

Internal examination

Before the days of reliable ultrasound, it was usual for doctors to perform an internal examination at the first antenatal visit. With the development of technology, however, this is now usually no longer routinely required.

Ultrasound scans

An ultrasound scan is usually performed at your first visit to confirm that the pregnancy is continuing and also to establish your estimated date of delivery. You are able to see your baby's heart beating on the scan and sometimes you can see movements even before you can feel them. The scan provides important additional information, such as whether or not there is an ovarian cyst and if you are due to have twins (see opposite page).

A scan is often repeated at 11–16 weeks to confirm the stage of the pregnancy. A so-called 'detailed' or 'anomaly' scan is often offered at 18–20 weeks to check if the baby has any abnormality (see page 147).

In later pregnancy, you might require further scans if the doctor is concerned that a problem is developing or wants to check on the baby's growth. The site of the placenta can also be assessed and the lie and presentation of the baby if these are hard to determine by clinical examination. Ultrasound is routinely used to check the growth of twins as it is impossible to assess their size accurately by examination alone.

Twins

A twin pregnancy occurs spontaneously in around 1:80 conceptions. There are two sorts of twins: non-identical or fraternal twins (referred to as dizygotic twins), and identical twins (referred to as monozygotic twins). Non-identical twins occur when the mother produces two eggs and both are fertilized and implanted in the womb successfully. The likelihood of non-identical twins is increased in assisted conception techniques (see pages 87–111).

By contrast, identical twins occur following the splitting of a single fertilized egg. The egg effectively splits into two after fertilization and two identical children develop. Identical twins are less common than non-identical twins. There is a marked variation throughout the world in the chance of having non-identical twins. This ranges from between 2 and 7 per 1,000 births in Japan and China, to between 8 and 20 per 1,000 in Europe and the USA to more than 20 per 1,000 births in Nigeria and Jamaica. In addition, non-identical twins have a familial factor which can be passed from mother to daughter, making you more likely to have non-identical twins if your mother had twins.

must know

Twin complications
There is an increased risk of complications in a twin pregnancy, including miscarriage, abnormalities in the babies, pre-eclampsia, small-for-dates babies, anaemia and premature labour. Twin pregnancies tend to go into labour at around three weeks in advance of singleton pregnancies.

Screening for abnormalities

While the majority of pregnancies result in healthy babies, a small proportion of babies are born with an abnormality. These can be very minor problems, such as a small skin tag, or a major problem like spina bifida or Down's syndrome.

Determining an abnormality

Doctors now have the ability to determine if your baby is affected by certain serious abnormalities. Two approaches are taken to try to identify babies that might have a serious abnormality: screening tests and diagnostic tests. Screening tests can be applied to large numbers of women. They don't give a definite answer as to whether your baby has an abnormality but provide an indication of your level of risk for a particular abnormality. For example, a screening test for Down's syndrome might give you a risk of 1:1,000 for the baby having Down's syndrome. This would be a low risk; while it does not guarantee absolutely that the baby will not be affected, it obviously would be extremely unlikely. Conversely, the screening test might give a result of 1:50, which would be a relatively high risk, but again does not mean that the baby is affected. Indeed, there are 49 chances out of 50 that it won't be. So screening tests help to show which mothers are more likely to have a problem, but don't provide a definite answer.

Where a definite answer is needed, a diagnostic test is used. Here a sample of fluid, blood or tissue is taken from the womb, placenta or umbilical cord, as in amniocentesis where a sample of amniotic fluid is removed. Because such tests are invasive, they carry a risk to the pregnancy (see page 145), but a definite diagnosis can be obtained so that you know for sure whether or not your baby is affected by a specific condition like Down's syndrome. The table opposite outlines the screening and diagnostic tests that are available.

Feelings on diagnosis of an abnormality

How you may feel very much depends on your wishes and the severity of the abnormality. Some abnormalities, like cleft lip, can be easily corrected by surgery after the baby is born. Other conditions, like severe spina bifida and hydrocephalus, might be very disabling or even fatal for the baby. In these instances, doctors usually offer you a termination of the pregnancy. However, only you can decide the right course of action for you. You will probably need time to consider the options and get more information on the condition and what it would mean for you and your baby. The decision is yours and doctors and midwives are there to help give you accurate information and answer your questions.

Screening tests

Test	When is it done?	What does it tell you?
Nuchal (neck) translucency scan	10–14 weeks	Down's syndrome risk, may be combined with the double or triple test (below)
Double or triple blood test	15–20 weeks (ideally 15–18 weeks)	Risk of neural tube defect and Down's syndrome

Diagnostic tests

Test	When is it done?	What does it tell you?
Chorionic villous sampling (CVS) (sample of tissue taken from the placenta)	9–12 weeks	Identifies genetic problems like Down's syndrome
Amniocentesis (sample of fluid taken from the womb)	15–18 weeks	Identifies genetic problems like Down's syndrome
Cordocentesis (blood sample taken from the umbilical cord)	From 18 weeks	Identifies genetic abnormalities or problems like viral infection and severe anaemia
Detailed ultrasound scan	18–20 weeks	Identifies structural abnormalities like spina bifida and cleft lip

Screening tests

Whether or not you have any of these tests is entirely your own choice. Some women are happy to accept the outcome of the pregnancy no matter what, while others want the reassurance of screening tests and some who might be at high risk want a diagnostic test. This is a personal issue and your views should determine what tests, if any, are carried out. Ask your doctor or midwife who will be able to advise you.

must know

Nuchal scan accuracy
This test is by no means 100 per cent accurate. It aims to identify babies who are more likely to have a problem. It is often combined with the blood tests that also screen for this problem.

Nuchal translucency scan

Nuchal means 'neck', so a nuchal scan looks at the baby's neck. This is a fairly new technique that has been introduced to help screen for Down's syndrome and can be performed at around 10–14 weeks. Babies with Down's syndrome have a thicker pad of fat at the back of their neck than babies without the condition.

Double or triple blood test

The most widely used screening tests on blood samples are for spina bifida (and other neural tube defects) and Down's syndrome. This blood test is usually offered between 15 and 20 weeks. Obviously it is best to get the test done as early as possible as further investigations might be required.

The test measures three key substances in your blood. For this reason it is often called the 'triple test', although some centres use only two of the three measurements, in which case it is called the 'double test'. The substances that are measured in the triple test are all produced by the placenta and consist of:

- alpha-fetoprotein (AFP)
- oestriol
- human chorionic gonadotrophin (hCG)

In cases of spina bifida, AFP is increased, whereas in cases of Down's syndrome there is a reduction of both AFP and oestriol, while hCG is actually elevated.

If you are found to have an increased risk of spina bifida, you will be offered a detailed ultrasound scan to look specifically at the baby's back and head. If there is an increased risk of Down's syndrome, assessment of the risk may be modified via a nuchal scan. If the risk of Down's syndrome is considered high, you will be offered a diagnostic test, such as amniocentesis (see page 143).

Diagnostic tests

This kind of testing is essential to establish whether the developing baby has certain conditions that can be tested for. Information to confirm the diagnosis may only be obtained by carrying out so-called 'invasive' tests. They carry a risk of complications, so you must weigh up the risks of the test against the risk of the baby having the particular problem that you are testing for. Chorionic villous sampling (CVS) and amniocentesis can disturb the womb or placenta and trigger a miscarriage. The pregnancy loss rate associated with CVS is one to two per cent and for amniocentesis, it is about one per cent. Many women wait for the result of screening tests like the triple test or nuchal scan before deciding on whether or not they want an amniocentesis.

must know

Down's syndrome
The risk of having a baby with Down's syndrome increases with the age of the mother. At the age of 40, the chances of having a baby with Down's syndrome is around 1:100 compared to around 1:400 at the age of 36 and 1:1,000 at the age of 20 years.

Chorionic villus sampling (CVS)
The benefit of CVS is that it can be performed at 9–12 weeks and hence identify a problem earlier than can be done via amniocentesis. The chorionic villi are little fingers of tissue that form part of the placenta. As the placenta has the same genetic make-up as the foetus, this tissue can be used for the diagnosis of genetic and chromosomal problems. With CVS, a needle is inserted through the abdomen and into the edge of the placenta. This is done under ultrasound control so that the doctor can guide the needle to the site of the placenta. A tiny sample of chorionic villus tissue is then sucked up the needle using a syringe and the tissue is sent to the laboratory so that the genetic make-up of the baby can be ascertained: its sex and whether or not it has Down's syndrome or suffers from a genetic disease like cystic fibrosis. It can usually take up to three weeks to get the final result although sometimes a more rapid result can be obtained.

Amniocentesis
Amniocentesis is a procedure used to obtain a small amount of the amniotic fluid from around the unborn baby and is usually carried out at 15–18 weeks of the pregnancy. You are offered an amniocentesis if you are over 35 years of age or if the blood test for Down's syndrome or a nuchal scan shows you are at increased risk. You might also be offered an amniocentesis if you have a family history of a genetic disease and you want to know if the baby is affected by it.

Under local anaesthetic, a fine needle is inserted through the skin on your abdomen and into your womb. Ultrasound is used so that the doctor can see where the needle is going and avoid hitting the placenta or the baby. The needle is inserted into a pool of fluid in the womb and 10–15 ml (about three teaspoonfuls) of amniotic fluid is withdrawn by attaching a syringe to the end of the needle. This fluid contains some of the baby's cells, which are then grown in the laboratory. The same results can be determined as for testing with CVS.

Ultrasound scan

Ultrasound is one of the best ways to check that an unborn baby appears to be developing normally. By 18–20 weeks the baby is well developed and big enough to allow all the major parts of its anatomy to be seen on an ultrasound scan. The sex of the baby can usually be determined, too. Many obstetricians now offer scans at this stage to check for any abnormality, referred to as detailed or anomaly scans.

Ultrasound can be used for both screening and diagnosis. The types of abnormality that can be diagnosed by ultrasound include neural tube defects like spina bifida and hydrocepahalus, major heart defects, abdominal wall defects, bladder problems, abnormalities of the limbs and cleft lip and palate.

did you know?

Screening and diagnosis
Ultrasound was pioneered by a Glaswegian obstetrician, Professor Ian Donald in Glasgow, in the late 1950s. In under half a century ultrasound has revolutionized not only pregnancy care, but also in the diagnosis of many conditions, from heart disease and blood clots in the leg, to gallstones.

6 Facing problems

Women who have a pre-existing medical condition, such as diabetes or epilepsy, often face specific issues in pregnancy linked to their condition or the drugs used to treat it. So it is important to consider the effects of the condition and its associated medication on the pregnancy, and also the effect of pregnancy on the medical condition.

Complications caused by pregnancy

Although many pregnancies go smoothly, many others have complications. In early pregnancy, miscarriage is a relatively common problem and occasionally there is an ectopic pregnancy. In late pregnancy, specific conditions can occur, such as pre-eclampsia. These three areas are covered in this section.

Ectopic pregnancy

An ectopic pregnancy occurs when the fertilized egg implants in a location other than the womb. This happens in around 1:300 pregnancies. The most common site for ectopic pregnancy is a fallopian tube as over 95 per cent of implants occur there. However, implant can also occur at the junction of the tube and the womb, on the ovaries, in the abdomen or even on the cervix. As the fallopian tube is not designed to allow a pregnancy to develop, the tube will eventually rupture as the pregnancy grows. This will lead to serious bleeding inside the abdomen, which can be life threatening. It is unusual for a tubal pregnancy to proceed beyond eight to ten weeks – either it will perish and resolve itself or lead to symptoms indicating the need for medical intervention.

Why ectopic pregnancies occur

Ectopic pregnancy is becoming increasingly common in the West, with a several-fold increase over the last 20 years. This is due to an increasing incidence of pelvic inflammatory disease, causing infection of the womb and fallopian tubes and leading to tubal damage, in addition to the effects on the tubes of surgery, including sterilization and its reversal. Such damage to the fallopian tubes can slow the progress of the fertilized egg as it journeys down the tube to the womb. If this process is delayed, the pregnancy implants in the tube.

In addition, the rising incidence of ectopic pregnancy may reflect improvements in diagnosis of the problem. There are now very highly sensitive pregnancy tests and high-quality ultrasound scans that can identify a pregnancy at a much earlier stage than was possible years ago. This allows the early identification of ectopic pregnancies that in the past may have resolved without any treatment and before they became a clinical problem.

Diagnosing an ectopic pregnancy

If you have an ectopic pregnancy, the most common signs are pain in the lower abdomen, usually on one side, and vaginal bleeding in early pregnancy. The pain may be present over several days or come on suddenly. Occasionally there is pain in the shoulder tip. Because of the serious implications of ectopic pregnancy, you must see a doctor urgently if you have any of these symptoms.

The two key features in the diagnosis are to confirm that you are pregnant (through a pregnancy test) and to determine whether the pregnancy is inside the womb (through an ultrasound scan). If you have a positive pregnancy test and there is no pregnancy in the womb, the pregnancy must be somewhere else and must therefore be an ectopic pregnancy.

Sometimes it is difficult to distinguish an ectopic pregnancy from a very early pregnancy that is in the

must know
Future fertility
An ectopic pregnancy damages the fallopian tube and will inevitably affect future fertility. Unfortunately, over half of women who have had an ectopic pregnancy will have difficulty in becoming pregnant again without assisted conception (see page 87–111) and 12–18 per cent of women who have had an ectopic pregnancy will have a further ectopic pregnancy.

did you know?

Early detection
Ultrasound scans performed through the vagina, rather than the abdomen, provide a better image in early pregnancy and therefore better potential for early detection of ectopic pregnancy.

womb. With a normal pregnancy in the womb, the concentration of hCG in the blood doubles approximately every two days and this can be measured by taking several blood samples. In an ectopic pregnancy, however, the doubling rate is much slower. There is also a level of hCG at which a pregnancy would definitely be seen in the womb using ultrasound. If this level has been reached and no pregnancy is seen in the womb, then the pregnancy must be ectopic.

Treating an ectopic pregnancy

The classic treatment of ectopic pregnancy is using surgery. The abdomen is opened and the fallopian tube with the ectopic pregnancy is removed to arrest or prevent serious bleeding as a result of its rupturing. Increasingly, doctors are leaving the tube in place if it has not ruptured. Although the tube is damaged, future prospects for a successful pregnancy may still be more favourable if the tube is left in place. 'Keyhole' surgery is also used to deal with ectopic pregnancy, which allows a faster recovery and shorter time in hospital than conventional surgery and might reduce the risk of a further ectopic pregnancy.

Sometimes ectopic pregnancy will not require any surgery. If you are clinically stable and at a very early stage in pregnancy with a small unruptured ectopic pregnancy, then sometimes doctors will simply monitor you to determine whether any specific treatment is necessary. Some early ectopic pregnancies may end without leading to haemorrhage or tubal rupture. Treatment with drugs to stop the pregnancy growing is also being explored.

Miscarriage

A miscarriage is the spontaneous loss of a pregnancy before the 24th week. When the fetus is younger than 24 weeks, it is generally not capable of sustaining life outside its mother. The vast majority of miscarriages occur before weeks ten to twelve of pregnancy. Many women worry about the possibility of having a miscarriage, especially if they have had one before. There are a couple of things that you should know.

First of all, miscarriages occur in up to 15 per cent of all clinically confirmed pregnancies. There are several known causes of miscarriage, but despite this, doctors can often find no cause and the majority of miscarriages remain unexplained, though at least some may be 'nature's way' of dealing with a problem in the pregnancy. In this situation, there is usually nothing that anyone can do, particularly you, to prevent a miscarriage. So, if you have a miscarriage, try not take on responsibility for it occurring.

Second, some bleeding in early pregnancy does not always lead to a miscarriage. There is an unfounded myth that you may still have a period when you are pregnant – any bleeding that occurs in early pregnancy cannot be due to a period. The main problem associated with bleeding in early pregnancy is threatened or actual miscarriage, although it is important to exclude ectopic pregnancy (see opposite). Occasionally, bleeding may come from a lesion at the neck of the womb, such as a polyp, a fold of tissue on the skin that bleeds easily, but this will not affect the pregnancy.

must know

Causes of bleeding in early pregnancy
- threatened miscarriage
- complete or incomplete miscarriage
- ectopic pregnancy
- bleeding from the neck of the womb (cervix), such as from a polyp

The known causes of miscarriage

Abnormal-shaped womb Examples of an abnormal-shaped womb are a bicornuate uterus, where instead of having a triangular cavity the womb is shaped in the form of two 'horns', or a unicornuate uterus where the womb is shaped like a single horn. However, many women with these abnormalities have successful pregnancies so it is difficult to establish whether this is a genuine cause of miscarriage or just a coincidental finding.

Genetic abnormalities 'Mistakes' in the genetic blueprint for development may arise at around the time of conception and are a common cause of miscarriage. Such mistakes can mean that the pregnancy will not succeed as the pregnancy does not have the correct genetic information to develop properly.

Hormonal disturbance Disturbance of the levels of hormones controlling ovulation and early pregnancy has been linked to miscarriage, but correcting these problems does not appear to prevent miscarriages from happening.

Infection An infection within the womb or affecting the fetus can lead to miscarriage, but this is very uncommon. Most of the common causes of vaginal discharge in pregnancy, such as thrush, are not associated with miscarriage.

Medical conditions A medical condition in the mother can sometimes cause miscarriage, such as untreated thyroid disease, poorly controlled diabetes, chronic kidney disease and conditions where the mother has a tendency to form blood clots that can damage the placenta.

Weak cervix (neck of the womb) Until labour occurs, the cervix must remain tightly closed to keep the baby safely in the womb and to prevent any infection reaching the developing baby. Weakness of the cervix, known as 'cervical incompetence', may be due to a problem that you are born with, or can be due to the cervix being damaged during surgery or childbirth. With cervical incompetence, recurrent miscarriage will occur, with minimal pain. Usually the womb has to contract powerfully, and very painfully, to deliver the baby. With cervical incompetence, the cervix opens without contractions – hence the absence of pain. Miscarriage because of cervical incompetence will initially be in the middle of pregnancy, with subsequent miscarriages occurring earlier and earlier. The condition is treatable by a special stitch to keep the neck of the womb closed.

Vaginal bleeding in early pregnancy
If this happens to you, call your GP or the hospital immediately, particularly if pain is associated with the bleeding. Because suspected miscarriages are so common, many hospitals have specialized early-pregnancy assessment units, usually staffed with specially trained doctors and midwives, which can provide rapid assessment and management of problems in early pregnancy problems. Often this is carried out on an outpatient basis.

To find out what is happening, the doctor will ask you certain questions, examine you and usually arrange an ultrasound scan within 24 hours. It can sometimes also be useful to repeat your pregnancy test. The doctor will be trying to establish several key pieces of information:

- Confirm that you are definitely pregnant.
- Confirm that your pregnancy is within the womb (and not ectopic).
- Determine whether your pregnancy is still viable via an ultrasound test.
- Determine how far advanced your pregnancy is.
- Establish when the bleeding occurred; for example, whether it came on after intercourse, suggesting a local problem such as a polyp.
- Establish how heavy your bleeding was, whether there was any pain and whether any tissue was passed along with the blood.
- Find out whether you have had miscarriages before. It is unusual to find a cause for miscarriage in a woman who has had a single miscarriage. However, women with recurrent miscarriages are often found to have an underlying cause and should therefore be investigated. Some causes of recurrent miscarriage can be successfully treated.

The different types of miscarriage

Name	Symptoms	What happens
Threatened miscarriage	Painless vaginal bleeding from the site of the placenta in your womb.	The bleeding is often not severe enough to trouble the pregnancy; it can settle and the pregnancy may continue normally. When you are examined, the cervix is closed. Sometimes a threatened miscarriage will lead to an inevitable miscarriage.
Inevitable miscarriage	Severe 'cramping' pain caused by contractions, accompanying bleeding.	The cervix is usually open due to uterine contractions attempting to expel the pregnancy from the womb.
Complete miscarriage	An inevitable miscarriage may progress to a complete miscarriage.	The whole pregnancy has been expelled from the womb and so the uterus is empty. With a complete miscarriage, the cervix is usually closed.
Incomplete miscarriage	Alternatively, an inevitable miscarriage may progress to an incomplete miscarriage.	Part of the embryo or fetus has been expelled from the womb but there is some tissue remaining. The cervix is usually found to be open due to the womb trying to expel the remaining pregnancy tissue.
Blighted ovum	Placental tissue develops in the womb but no embryo or fetus is found. There is no known reason for this failure of development, but the pregnancy obviously cannot continue and a blighted ovum will eventually progress to an inevitable miscarriage and, in turn, to an incomplete or complete miscarriage.	Serial ultrasound scans through the vagina at six weeks or earlier, at least one week apart, are used to confirm that no embryo is developing. It is important that serial ultrasound scans are carried out in case the dates of the pregnancy are wrong. If the pregnancy is earlier than thought, the ultrasound findings could be misinterpreted.

Name	Symptoms	What happens
Missed miscarriage (sometimes called a delayed miscarriage)	With a missed miscarriage there is usually no pain or bleeding. Often you will have stopped feeling pregnant. This will eventually progress to an inevitable miscarriage and, in turn, to an incomplete or complete miscarriage.	Diagnosed via ultrasound, the embryo or fetus is seen but the fetal heart is not beating, indicating that the pregnancy has ended some time before. Should the size of the embryo be consistent with a very early stage in pregnancy (in which the heartbeat wouldn't be detectable), the scan is repeated to confirm that no change has occurred, in case the menstrual dates are inaccurate.
The vanishing twin	A twin pregnancy is identified on an initial scan early in pregnancy, and a subsequent scan shows only one baby.	One of the twins may have been miscarried or even reabsorbed into the placenta, while the other twin continues to develop in the womb without any apparent problems.

Treating miscarriage

Threatened miscarriage is treated by nothing more specific than reassurance and follow-up ultrasound scans to check that everything is going well. There is no need to be admitted to hospital or confined to bed, although it is sensible to avoid excessive physical stress.

Following a complete miscarriage, the possibility of an ectopic pregnancy will have to be discounted (see page 150-2). The treatment of complete miscarriage is reassurance – that miscarriage is common; it may not happen again; nothing could have been done to prevent it and no further action is needed.

In cases of incomplete miscarriage, blighted ovum and missed miscarriage, the pregnancy has ended and the treatment is to proceed to empty the womb either medically (with drugs) or surgically – a procedure known as 'evacuation of the uterus' (see below). Increasingly, 'expectant' management is offered, where doctors wait for the womb to contract and evacuate itself, while observing the situation with scans. It is important to ensure that your womb is empty, as dead tissue retained in the uterus can lead to bleeding and infection. Infection can cause you to become very ill, or even threaten your future fertility by damaging the fallopian tubes. If you have a miscarriage, should discuss the best management of it for you with your doctor.

must know

The chances of infection
Significant infection is uncommon with surgical, medical or expectant management – about two to three per cent with each.

Evacuation of the uterus (D&C)

Surgical evacuation of the uterus is usually carried out under general anaesthesia. Your cervix is often open following an incomplete miscarriage, which allows the surgeon access to the womb. If the cervix is not already open, it is gently stretched open using instruments called dilators. This can be made easier by the use of special pessaries given before the operation to soften the cervix before the dilatation. The wall of the womb may then be scraped with an instrument called a curette to ensure that it is empty and no pieces of tissue still adhere to the uterus. Drugs are given to make the womb contract as contractions minimize any bleeding during and after the evacuation.

An alternative to surgical evacuation, and more appropriate in certain cases such as missed miscarriage or incomplete miscarriage, is medical evacuation using drugs. Drugs are given that cause your womb to contract strongly so expelling any tissue. The womb can be checked with ultrasound after medical evacuation to ensure it is empty. If it is not empty, surgical evacuation may be required, but this is not often necessary.

Potential miscarriage complications

The most common complications that are encountered after miscarriage are haemorrhage and infection, both of which are often due to retained pregnancy tissue.

• In cases of severe haemorrhage, drugs are given to contract the womb and reduce bleeding while awaiting surgical evacuation.

• The risk of infection is reduced by prompt evacuation of the uterus to remove any remaining dead tissue, which acts as a fertile breeding ground for bacteria. Infection can cause you to have abdominal and pelvic pain and tenderness, a high temperature, and often an offensive vaginal discharge. In addition, it can sometimes cause heavy bleeding from the womb.

If there is a possibility of infection in the womb, the doctor takes bacteriological swabs from any discharge at the top of the vagina and the inside of the cervix. The swabs are sent to the bacteriology laboratory for analysis to determine what, if any, bacteria are causing the infection. Antibiotics suitable for dealing with the majority of bacteria that cause infection in the womb should be given as soon as possible.

Emotions following a miscarriage

Inevitably, many women, and their partners, feel completely devastated and heartbroken after a miscarriage. The majority describe feeling that a part of them has died. The loss of a pregnancy is therefore a very distressing experience. More than half of all women suffering a miscarriage want something to remember their baby by, such as an ultrasound scan photograph. Often women feel they have failed or have a sense of guilt or anxiety. Others react with anger. These are all normal reactions to grief and bereavement. Many women feel a sense of loneliness after a miscarriage. Anxiety about the ability to conceive successfully in the future, and indeed persisting through subsequent pregnancies, is common. A great deal of support is therefore required, not just after a miscarriage but also in any future pregnancy.

Depression is common after a miscarriage and the emotional problems can cause difficulties in relationships. Patience, understanding and support from partners is required. It is important to talk about the problem with partners, families or friends. Some women find it especially useful to discuss the situation with someone who has experienced a similar problem or someone who can explain how miscarriages occur and answer the questions that arise. The appropriate emotional support varies from woman to woman; however, there are several support groups to turn to. Your GP or obstetrician and gynecologist can also provide specific medical information and support for you at this time.

Almost three-quarters of women worry that they might have caused the problem leading to their miscarriage. They think back on the pregnancy and try to identify something that they have done or not done which could have caused the problem. This is, at least partly, because doctors can usually give them no specific medical reason for the miscarriage. The truth, however, is that it is exceptionally rare for there to have been anything that the mother could have done or not done which would have caused or prevented the miscarriage. Knowing this may not alleviate the sense of loss or bereavement, but may help her understand that the miscarriage was not preventable and therefore not her responsibility.

Further pregnancies

From a physical point of view, it is usually reasonable to try to conceive after the menstrual cycle has returned to normal following an uncomplicated miscarriage. Perhaps more important to consider, however, is if you are ready emotionally to deal with another pregnancy. Only you and your partner can really determine this. If you have had a miscarriage, you should try and avoid pregnancy until you and your partner feel able to cope with the anxiety that a pregnancy will inevitably generate.

Recurring miscarriages

Miscarriages are common; they are the most common complication in pregnancy. So it is not unusual for a woman to have more than one. Indeed, recurrent miscarriage (the medical definition of

must know

Successful pregnancies

In many cases of recurrent miscarriage, no cause is found. However, while this is unsatisfactory in terms of explaining the problem, it does not mean the situation is hopeless. In such cases, 75 per cent of women go on, with supportive care alone, to have a successful pregnancy.

recurrent miscarriage is the loss of three or more consecutive pregnancies) is a problem that affects around one per cent of women. Around five per cent of women will have two consecutive miscarriages. Although it is very unusual to be able identify a specific cause for a miscarriage, where recurrent miscarriages occur, it is important to perform investigations to exclude the known causes of recurrent miscarriage, some of which are treatable. Many doctors will not perform such investigations until three miscarriages have occurred, unless there are special considerations or a strong suspicion of an underlying medical problem.

In the first instance, the genetic make-up of the parents is checked (and, if possible, so is the pregnancy that miscarried), through a simple blood test. In fewer than five per cent of cases, one or other parent is shown to carry a genetic abnormality. It is also important to screen for specific medical conditions. In particular, 15 per cent of women with recurrent miscarriage have antiphospholipid antibody syndrome, a condition that predisposes the mother to develop blood clots that can damage the placenta and lead to pregnancy loss. This condition can be treated using drugs to prevent clotting. Another treatable cause of miscarriage is cervical incompetence, which is treated surgically with a stitch to support and reinforce the cervix.

Pre-eclampsia

Pre-eclampsia is a pregnancy complication found in two to three per cent of pregnancies. It can only occur in the second half of pregnancy and will resolve within a few weeks or months of delivery. It causes high blood pressure and kidney upset in the mother and can also

must know

Other potential complications

Pre-eclampsia can lead to impaired liver function and occasionally the blood-clotting system will be disturbed. You may also have a headache, blurred vision and see flashing lights, feel pain in your abdomen below your ribcage and sometimes vomit. In its most severe form, eclampsia, convulsions (fits) occur, due to the brain being upset by the condition.

disturb the baby's growth. Pre-eclampsia can be dangerous as there are no symptoms until it is very severe. That is why your blood pressure and urine are checked at every visit as the first signs of pre-eclampsia are picked up though an increase in your blood pressure or protein in your urine.

When pre-eclampsia might occur

The cause of pre-eclampsia is unknown. It seems chiefly due to the abnormal implantation of the placenta into the mother's womb, although it's not clear why this should occur. A signal appears to be released from the large placenta, which triggers the condition. The placenta may also not be sufficient to meet the baby's needs and could even restrict the baby's growth.

Treating pre-eclampsia

There is no proven treatment that can prevent pre-eclampsia. Low-dose aspirin (60–75 mg a day), which reduces the activity of certain parts of the clotting system, might be prescribed in some cases. This will reduce the risk of pre-eclampsia by about 15 per cent. This treatment is often started at the time of the first antenatal visit if you are considered to be at risk.

When it occurs, the aim of treatment is to protect the mother and the baby from the consequences of high blood pressure. Thus treatment with medication to control the blood pressure is often required. This allows the pregnancy to continue for as long as possible to try to avoid premature delivery. Your doctor will regularly weigh up the risk to the mother and baby of continuing with the pregnancy against the risks of complicated delivery.

did you know?
Pre-eclampsia is more likely if you:
• are in your first pregnancy
• usually have high blood pressure
• suffer from migraine
• have diabetes or kidney disease
• have already had pre-eclampsia
• are over 35 or less than 20 years of age
• are expecting twins
• have a family history of pre-eclampsia

Pre-existing medical problems

Many women have pre-existing medical problems – up to eight per cent of women have asthma, one to two per cent suffer from chronic high blood pressure, one per cent from epilepsy, a further one per cent from thyroid disease and so on. This adds up to a considerable number of women.

did you know?

Pre-existing medical condition

As your body adapts to pregnancy in order to meet the demands of the growing baby:
• your heart will increase the amount of blood that it pumps round your body every minute by about 40 per cent
• the blood flow to your kidneys increases in order to help them get rid of waste products in the urine, from both you and the baby, at a higher rate
• the amount of blood in your body increases and you will be making more red blood cells to carry oxygen round the body
• although you probably won't notice it, you will breathe more deeply and the amount of air passing in and out of your lungs may increase by as much as 40–50 per cent

These women with pre-existing medical problems can and do become pregnant and have successful deliveries. It is worth remembering, however, that many medical problems can influence your pregnancy and that pregnancy can have an effect on your medical condition. This is what this section focuses on. If you need to take regular medication, pregnancy can influence its effectiveness, while some medication can have potentially harmful effects on the unborn child. All of this is best weighed up before you embark on pregnancy.

If you have a medical condition or are on long-term drug therapy, discuss the implications of your condition, and any drugs used to treat it, with your doctor before conceiving and then their effect once you are pregnant. Some medication can be safely continued; other medication requires modification or discontinuation. Depending on the condition, you may require specialist help, which your doctor can usually arrange. This will allow optimal planning and treatment of your condition before and during pregnancy.

As this can be a complex issue, it is essential to seek medical advice prior to pregnancy, before altering any treatment. Ill-advised or unnecessary changes in treatment may precipitate problems not only for your baby, but also for your own health. Some of the more common medical conditions are discussed in this chapter.

Asthma

Asthma commonly affects up to eight per cent of young women, so it is not unusual for it to be encountered in pregnancy, which has a variable affect on asthma. In some women, the asthma worsens and in others, it stays the same, while there are others in whom it improves.

What happens in pregnancy

Until you are pregnant it is generally impossible to predict what will happen, although it is unusual for a mother with well-controlled asthma and minimal symptoms to develop significant problems in pregnancy in the absence of some other complicating factor, such as a bad chest infection. However, women with severe asthma may find it gets worse in the later stages of pregnancy when the womb is very large and so can affect breathing. While well-controlled asthma is very unlikely to affect your pregnancy, uncontrolled severe asthma can be associated with low oxygen levels in your blood, which could potentially upset the baby. This is very uncommon.

None of the medications commonly used to treat asthma pose any significant risk to the baby. Indeed, the risks posed by uncontrolled asthma far outweigh the risks associated with any of these medications. Furthermore, they are all safe to take while you are breastfeeding your baby.

watch out!

Oral steroid medication, especially at high doses, can mean there is an increased risk of developing gestational diabetes.

Treatment in pregnancy

• Treatment is virtually identical to treatment when you are not pregnant. If possible, avoid anything that you know triggers your asthma.

• You may need to monitor your peak flow. A 'dip' in your peak flow measurement, particularly in the evening, may precede worsening of your wheeze, and this can help you or your doctors adjust your therapy to prevent your symptoms getting worse.

• In labour, continue your usual asthma medication. If you have been on steroid tablets, you may need some steroid injections, too. Your doctor will advise you about this. All the usual forms of pain relief are safe. However, if you need a Caesarean delivery, then epidural or spinal analgesia is better than a general anaesthetic.

Diabetes

Insulin is a hormone produced by the pancreas, a gland in the abdomen, and is essential for regulating blood-sugar levels. When your pancreas produces insufficient insulin, blood-sugar levels rise and diabetes occurs.

What happens in pregnancy

If you have insulin-dependent diabetes, you are at an increased risk of pregnancy complications, which can affect both you and your baby. There is a small increase in the risk of congenital abnormalities in the baby, such as cleft palate, heart and kidney abnormalities, and neural tube defects like spina bifida. This risk is about three times higher than that of a non-diabetic mother and appears to be related to high levels of glucose (sugar) in the blood in early pregnancy, at the time that the baby's organs are forming.

Miscarriage is also more common in women with poorly controlled diabetes. In addition, the baby is at risk of being large, due in part to the excess sugar it may receive, which can lead to problems in labour and delivery. It is not unusual for the baby to have excess fluid around it in the womb, making your womb large for dates. Often the doctor will monitor the baby's growth with ultrasound scans throughout the pregnancy. Diabetes puts you at increased risk of problems like pre-eclampsia. You will also be a little more prone to bladder infections and thrush.

Treatment in pregnancy

Women with diabetes frequently do become pregnant and have successful, untroubled pregnancies. Equally, pregnancy does not necessarily make diabetes worse, but your insulin requirements and your blood-sugar regulation will need to be altered.

There are special clinics for pregnant women with diabetes, with an obstetrician and a diabetic physician in attendance. There may also be specialist support from other professions, such as dietitians or midwives with an interest in diabetes. These clinics have been shown to be highly effective in managing diabetes in pregnancy.

• In pregnancy, hormones produced by the placenta have an anti-insulin effect, which can increase your insulin requirements. It is therefore important that insulin-dependent diabetic women have their condition well under control before conception.

• You will also be advised to take folic acid supplements to reduce the risk of fetal abnormality.

• You may be offered a blood test at around 16 weeks and a detailed ultrasound scan at 18–20 weeks to check for any abnormality in the baby. Your doctor will check

watch out!
If you suffer from morning sickness, it is critically important to maintain a reasonable intake of glucose (glucose-rich drinks can be helpful) and maintain your insulin treatment. In addition, try the usual remedies for morning sickness (see pages 116–9). Do not hesitate to get medical advice.

regularly for complications like urinary tract infection and pre-eclampsia and also carefully assess the baby's rate of growth.

• By the end of your pregnancy, your insulin requirements will have risen to two to three times that of your pre-pregnancy requirements. This is because of changes in the hormones that influence your blood-glucose control. After delivery of the placenta, your insulin requirements generally return to those of pre-pregnancy.

• Because there may be risks for the baby from going beyond the due date, most doctors try to deliver women with diabetes by their due date and often a little earlier.

Inheriting diabetes

There is no evidence that diabetes in pregnancy has any harmful effects in the long term on your child's intelligence or development. If your partner does not suffer from diabetes, there is a 2:100 chance of your child developing insulin-dependent diabetes before the age of 20. Where only the father has insulin-dependent diabetes, the baby has around a 1:20 chance of developing diabetes in later life – higher than if only the mother is affected!

Epilepsy

Epilepsy occurs in about 1:150 women, so it is not unusual for women with epilepsy to become pregnant. The majority of women with epilepsy will have a successful pregnancy with a healthy baby at the end of it, but there is a higher risk of certain antenatal complications.

There is about a four per cent chance of your baby being affected by epilepsy. However, if both you and your partner have epilepsy, then the chance of the baby developing epilepsy increases to about 2:10. The risk can vary according to the type of epilepsy that you have. Your own doctor can advise you about this.

What happens in pregnancy

In most women, there is no change in the frequency of seizures when they are pregnant. But around 25 per cent do find that the number of seizures they have increases, which is more likely if their epilepsy is not well controlled prior to pregnancy. Overall, the change in frequency is unpredictable and will not necessarily follow the pattern in a previous pregnancy.

Some of these increases in the frequency of fits may be due to women deliberately not taking their anti-epileptic medication as they worry that the drug will cause an abnormality in the baby, such as a neural tube defect like spina bifida. In any case, they usually stop their therapy too late to make a difference. The neural tube is formed seven weeks following the last period, so stopping medication after that time cannot prevent this abnormality and will only increase the risk of seizures, which in itself can cause problems.

Other reasons that seizures may increase are:
• if you have morning sickness and can't keep your medication down
• tiredness towards the end of pregnancy because it is often difficult to get a good night's sleep
• pregnancy can affect the levels of anti-epileptic medication in your blood. If there is an increase in the number of fits, your doctor might advise an increase in dose, provided you have been reliably taking the medication

There is a higher incidence of fetal abnormalities in babies of diabetic women possibly because of the folic

watch out!
There is no evidence that a single fit will cause the baby any problem. However, if you have a prolonged series of fits, this can be dangerous for both you and the baby. Fortunately, this is uncommon, but it indicates the importance of taking your anti-epileptic medication during pregnancy.

acid metabolism being upset by the anti-epileptic medication, although genetic factors might also play a part. It is therefore especially important for women on anti-epileptic medication to take folic acid when planning a pregnancy and to continue this in early pregnancy. The abnormalities most commonly seen are cleft lip and palate, heart defects and neural tube defects like spina bifida. Minor abnormalities like club foot can also occur. There is also an increased risk of pregnancy complications, like severe morning sickness, anaemia, vaginal bleeding and of having a baby that is small for dates.

Treatment in pregnancy

• No anti-epileptic medication is known to be totally free of risk, but risks increase when multiple anti-epileptic drugs are used. The risk of fetal abnormality ranges from around six per cent of women on one anti-epileptic drug to over 20 per cent in women on four drugs. The rate of abnormality is usually two to three per cent in women without epilepsy. Wherever possible, it is best if your epilepsy is controlled with one drug alone.

• You should see your doctor, who can advise you if your therapy needs to be changed. You might even want to have your medication reviewed prior to conception. Do not stop or alter your treatment without first consulting your doctor, or you may place yourself at increased risk of seizures, which can be harmful to you and your developing baby.

• Abnormalities that can occur in babies of women who suffer from epilepsy can be screened for during pregnancy. The good news is that the majority of

watch out!

Some anti-epileptic medications antagonize vitamin K, which is important for the production of clotting factors that stop us bleeding. Your doctor may therefore prescribe vitamin K tablets from around 36 weeks. These will boost not only your own but also your baby's vitamin K level.

babies born to mothers with epilepsy are not born with any abnormality.

Heart disease

Most women in the UK with heart disease will know before they get pregnant that they have a heart problem. The condition will usually have been treated and controlled long before they think about pregnancy. It is important, however, to determine how severe the problem is. Heart disease is often graded on the basis of the New York Heart Association classification of severity (see table, below). Regardless of the cause of heart problems, women with grades I or II symptoms are unlikely to have major problems during a pregnancy. Nonetheless, it is important if you have a heart problem and are considering pregnancy to obtain specific advice about your own situation. Your doctor should be able to advise you.

Severity of heart problems (after the New York Heart Association classification)

Grade I	No breathlessness and no problem with ordinary physical exercise
Grade II	No problem at rest but slight limitation of activities, such as walking, due to breathlessness
Grade III	Marked limitation of physical activity although no cardiac symptoms at rest
Grade IV	Breathlessness at rest

High blood pressure

Around three per cent of women have chronic high blood pressure before they become pregnant. This high blood pressure is known as 'hypertension' and in 90 per cent of cases it is due to so-called 'essential hypertension'. The causes of essential hypertension aren't known, but it does tend to run in families. This is one of the reasons why doctors ask if you have a family history of high blood pressure. Other medical conditions, such as kidney disorders, can also cause high blood pressure, but this is much less common than essential hypertension.

What happens in pregnancy

High blood pressure is associated with an increased risk of having pre-eclampsia (see pages 162–3) and a small-for-dates baby (one that has not grown as big as it should have for the stage it has reached in pregnancy) so you will require a little more antenatal care. There will need to be careful assessments of your blood pressure and urine at each antenatal check. The baby's growth will also be monitored. However, the majority of women with high blood pressure will go on to have a successful pregnancy. It is very unusual for pregnancy itself to change the outlook dramatically for women with essential hypertension.

Treatment in pregnancy

• If you take anti-hypertensive medication, this needs to be reviewed so you can avoid medication that may have harmful effects on the pregnancy. This is obviously best considered prior to pregnancy

must know

Safe medication
If you are on medication for high blood pressure and want to conceive, check with your doctor that the medication is safe to use in pregnancy. Some common and very effective blood pressure medications used can pose problems for the developing baby. You should switch to other types of medication with the advice of your doctor, to those which are known to be safe before, very early on and during pregnancy.

and you should consult your doctor when you are planning to conceive.

• Normally, blood pressure falls in the first half of pregnancy and this same reduction occurs in most women with essential hypertension. Your doctor may therefore be able to stop your blood pressure medication for part of the pregnancy.

• In mothers at high risk, low doses of aspirin are sometimes used to try to prevent pre-eclampsia from occurring.

Inflammatory bowel disease

There are two forms of inflammatory bowel disease: Crohn's disease and ulcerative colitis. These conditions together affect just over 1:1,000 young women. When uncontrolled, they cause symptoms such as diarrhoea, abdominal pain and weight loss. They may even require surgery if complications arise.

What happens in pregnancy

Pregnancy does not usually cause any worsening of inflammatory bowel disease. While a flare-up of ulcerative colitis can occur in pregnancy, this is no more likely to happen during pregnancy than when you are not pregnant. Indeed, the risk is lower if the problem is well controlled when you conceive. For Crohn's disease, the majority of women do not experience any worsening of their condition during pregnancy. Nor is the risk of pregnancy complications significantly altered where inflammatory bowel disease is well controlled before conception and throughout pregnancy. So it is best to conceive when the problem is well controlled and inactive.

If you have had surgery for inflammatory bowel disease, this sometimes has to be taken into account when considering the best way for you to deliver. Your doctor will be able to advise you about this.

Treatment in pregnancy
• The medications most commonly used to control inflammatory bowel disease, such as steroids, are considered safe for pregnancy and breastfeeding, but review your medication with your doctor when you are planning to conceive.
• In addition, it is usual for your doctor to recommend that you take folic acid vitamin supplements before and during pregnancy.

Irritable bowel syndrome (IBS)

IBS is a relatively common condition in women. With IBS there is an alteration of the bowel's mobility, which leads to recurrent episodes of abdominal pain due to bowel spasm, and altered bowel habit that can either be constipation or diarrhoea. Indeed, the constipation and diarrhoea may alternate. The cause of IBS isn't known, but it is associated with a diet low in roughage and high in refined carbohydrates. Symptoms can be triggered or worsened by stress. Although distressing, uncomfortable and sometimes debilitating during attacks, the symptoms of IBS do not cause any long-term serious harm. Most women with IBS will have been diagnosed with the problem before their pregnancy.

What happens in pregnancy
Because pregnancy can reduce the bowel's mobility, making you more prone to constipation, women who

have constipation as a major symptom of their IBS may find it gets worse. However, this will not harm the pregnancy.

Treatment in pregnancy
• The best treatment is a high-fibre diet. Your doctor can also give you medication to make your stools more bulky and this often helps relieve the symptoms.
• Sometimes medication to relieve bowel spasm can help, but you should not take any medication for this during pregnancy except on your doctor's advice.

Migraine

Migraine should be distinguished from more common tension headaches. Migraine causes a throbbing, one-sided headache. Indeed, the name migraine is derived from the Greek words 'hemi' and 'kranion', meaning 'half the skull', reflecting that the headache is on one side of the head only. The headache is often accompanied by sweating, nausea and vomiting and light tends to make the symptoms worse, so your natural instinct is to stay in a darkened room. Many women get warning of impending migraine as they get a visual disturbance with flashing lights or wavy lines. Sometimes strange sensations or ringing in the ear or a feeling of dizziness herald an attack.

What happens in pregnancy
The true mechanism of migraine is unknown, but it is related to changes in the blood vessels supplying the brain, which seem to open up more during an attack. Interestingly, women who suffer from migraine have a higher chance of developing pre-eclampsia in

pregnancy (see pages 162–3), although the link isn't fully understood. However, in over half of women who suffer from migraine, the condition actually improves during pregnancy.

Treatment in pregnancy
● Some of the medication used to treat and to prevent migraine attacks are not advised when you are pregnant, so consult your doctor before you get pregnant so that your therapy can be adjusted, if required. You should also source a suitable medication to treat an attack if you have one while pregnant.
● Paracetamol is not associated with any problems for the baby in pregnancy and so is safe to use for treatment although, again, you may wish to discuss this with your doctor.
● Some anti-nausea medications are also safe.
● For prevention of attacks, low doses of aspirin (60–75 mg) can be effective and there is good evidence from large trials that this has no harmful effect on the unborn child.

Multiple sclerosis (MS)

MS affects up to 1:1,000 of the population in the UK and tends to first present between the ages of 20 and 40. In this condition, the insulating material around nerve fibres is damaged, so upsetting the function of the nerves. While the cause of multiple sclerosis is unknown, it tends to be a relapsing and remitting condition with damage to the nerves occurring in different parts of the brain and nervous system at different times. Alternatively, it can be a chronic progressive disorder.

What happens in pregnancy

Women with MS can consider a pregnancy – their fertility is not usually affected. The condition is unlikely to present for the first time during pregnancy. A sufferer is also less likely to relapse during pregnancy. Those women whose bladders are affected may be prone to recurrent cystitis, so their urine is examined for infection at each antenatal check.

Almost half of women with MS experience a temporary worsening of their MS in the six months after delivery. However, there are no long-term detrimental effects of pregnancy or breastfeeding on its course. Similarly, MS tends not to have an effect on pregnancy or on the developing baby.

Treatment in pregnancy

• Sometimes antibiotics are prescribed to prevent recurrent bladder infections. If you take drugs for your MS, discuss this with your doctor before becoming pregnant.

Rheumatoid arthritis

People with rheumatoid arthritis suffer from painful, stiff and sometimes swollen joints. The hands and wrists are often affected and it is interestingly more common in women than in men and is found in 1–2:1,000 pregnancies.

What happens in pregnancy

Rheumatoid arthritis rarely causes significant problems in pregnancy, however, and indeed improves markedly during the course of the pregnancy in around 75 per cent of women. This may be due to increased production of anti-inflammatory steroid hormones by your body during pregnancy. Thus it is often possible during pregnancy to reduce the medication and sometimes no specific medication is needed at all. However, especially in women in whom the condition has improved during pregnancy, there is a risk of the rheumatoid arthritis worsening after the pregnancy is over.

Treatment in pregnancy
• Paracetamol is safe to use in pregnancy.
• Long-term use of non-steroidal anti-inflammatory drugs (NSAIDs) in pregnancy, however, can result in low levels of amniotic fluid around the baby, due to the baby's kidneys producing less urine. Hence doctors generally try to avoid using NSAIDs in pregnancy.
• Steroid therapy is usually considered safe in pregnancy although if it is used in high doses over a long period, the mother is at a greater risk of developing complications, such as gestational diabetes. If you are on steroids for more than a couple of weeks during pregnancy, you will usually need steroid injections when you are in labour. This will allow your body to cope better with the stress of labour.
• Discuss your medication with your doctor, ideally before you try to become pregnant.

Sickle-cell anaemia
Sickle-cell anaemia is an example of a genetic condition. You receive chromosomes from your mother and father and with them the genes that

make up your genetic code. A genetic condition is due to a mistake or mutation in the genetic code on a chromosome. This gene can be passed from parent to child. In sickle-cell anaemia, there is an abnormality in the gene controlling the formation of the red blood cells that carry oxygen around the body.

Some genetic conditions are 'dominant', others are 'recessive'. Sickle-cell anaemia is a recessive condition because for a baby to be affected it needs to inherit two sickle-cell genes, one from each parent. Each parent passes the gene to the child at conception. If one parent passes on the sickle-cell gene and the other passes on a normal gene, this is not sufficient to cause the condition. To pass on the two sickle-cell genes necessary to produce the disease, each parent has to be either affected by the disease themselves or be a carrier of it. A carrier has one normal gene and one abnormal gene. Carriers do not usually have the disease, but have the potential to pass this gene on to a child. They are unlikely to know that they have the gene unless there is a family history of the disease.

Occasionally the abnormal gene can be 'dominant', as in the case of brittle bone disease and Huntingtons chorea (in which brain cells degenerate, leading to jerky, involuntary movements and progressive dementia). This means that if the baby has one abnormal gene it is affected, even if the other gene is normal. In dominant conditions, only one parent need carry and pass on the gene. This doesn't just relate to disease, of course. Probably the most common example of a dominant gene is that for eye colour. The gene for brown eye-colour is dominant over the blue eye-colour gene.

So if a baby receives a 'blue' gene from her mother and a 'brown' gene from her father, she will have brown eyes. If she gets a 'blue' gene from both parents, she will have blue eyes.

Sickle-cell anaemia is a condition that affects the red blood cells and is most commonly found in people of African origin. It is so called because the red blood cells, which carry oxygen around the body, are crescent-shaped instead of their normal disc-shape. When there is a shortage of oxygen or when there is an infection in the body, these red blood cells clump together and so prevent the smooth flow of blood. As well as causing chronic anaemia, the condition can give rise to bone pain, kidney upset and lung problems. It may also increase the risk of thrombosis (blood clots). If you have sickle-cell anaemia or could be a carrier, it is important to discuss the implications of this with your doctor before becoming pregnant.

What happens in pregnancy
If you carry the trait – that is, you have one copy of the sickle-cell gene and one normal gene – you will not usually develop anaemia, but you will be more prone to kidney and bladder infections. Where there is a family history of the condition, have a blood test prior to getting pregnant to check whether you have sickle-cell trait. If you are found to be a carrier, your partner may wish to be tested prior to conception to see whether the baby would be likely to inherit sickle-cell disease.

Sickle-cell anaemia in the mother, where both copies of the mother's genes carry the sickling abnormality, carries a higher risk of giving birth to premature and low-birth weight babies.

Treatment in pregnancy

• During pregnancy, a woman with sickle-cell anaemia needs folic acid supplements and sometimes a blood transfusion.

• Iron supplements are not routinely required, however, and are only given when iron stores are low.

• Specialist antenatal care is needed as treatment has to be tailored to each woman's needs.

Systemic lupus erythematosis (SLE)

SLE affects roughly 1:1,000 women, but as it often occurs at around 25–35 years of age, it is therefore not unusual for women with SLE to be pregnant. SLE is an inflammatory condition that most often affects the joints and skin, and a rash over the cheeks is common, such as when you are exposed to sunlight. The kidneys can be involved and this can cause kidney damage and high blood pressure. Other organs like the lungs can sometimes be affected, too. It can also upset the blood, leading to problems like anaemia. The condition tends to come and go, with relapses and remissions.

What happens in pregnancy

SLE can be associated with particular problems in pregnancy, including miscarriage, premature delivery, a small-for-dates baby, pre-eclampsia and thrombosis. However, you are less likely to encounter these problems if you conceive when your SLE is not active and where any medication you are taking is minimal.

did you know?

Connective tissue disease

Connective tissue diseases are a group of conditions where inflammation attacks various parts of the body. Two examples of connective tissue disease are SLE (systemic lupus erythematosis) and rheumatoid arthritis. In rheumatoid arthritis it is the joints that are affected, while in SLE the joints, skin, kidneys and many other organs can be affected.

SLE is variable in its severity and in the problems it can cause. The particular problems you will be at risk of in pregnancy because of SLE will be determined by the severity of your condition, the particular organs involved, and by the level of key factors in your blood. What happened in any previous pregnancies will also be important.

Treatment in pregnancy

• The overriding concern regarding SLE when you are trying to get pregnant and also in pregnancy is to keep the disease from flaring up. The treatment of SLE in pregnancy therefore ideally requires collaboration between specialist physicians, obstetricians and pediatricians. It is best to discuss the problems of SLE in pregnancy with your doctors before you try to become pregnant.

• Regular monitoring of both you and the baby is required to check for problems like pre-eclampsia and impaired fetal growth. This means that you will usually be seen more frequently for antenatal checks and will have more frequent ultrasound scans to determine that the baby is growing well.

• Your doctor will also be watching for any evidence of a flare-up of your SLE. If one occurs, it will probably be managed with steroid medication. If you have high blood pressure, this should be controlled with suitable medication.

Thyroid problems

The thyroid gland helps control the body's metabolism. An overactive thyroid gland is known as hyper-thyroidism, the features of which include weight loss, palpitations, tremor, increased appetite, goitre (swelling of the thyroid gland in the neck), intolerance of heat and increased bowel function. This is a relatively common condition that is found in around 1:500 pregnancies.

An underactive thyroid gland is known as hypothyroidism and it affects around 1:100 women. The symptoms of hypothyroidism include tiredness, weight gain, constipation, hair loss, dry skin and very infrequent menstrual periods. It is usually identified and treated before pregnancy because, without treatment, you will be unlikely to conceive because of the effect on your periods.

What happens in pregnancy
Hyperthyroidism does not usually pose any special problems in pregnancy provided the condition is kept under control. If it is uncontrolled, there is a risk of problems like miscarriage, a small-for-dates baby and premature labour. It is also unusual for hypothyroidism to cause any significant problems in pregnancy.

Treatment in pregnancy
For hyperthyroidism:
• With medications, which do not cause any serious abnormalities in the baby, although you should follow your doctor's advice. These are safe for breastfeeding as only very small amounts are found in breast milk and do not appear to cause the baby any problem.
• The thyroid function is tested during pregnancy by a simple blood test, to make sure that the overactive thyroid is under control.
• Sometimes the doctor checks on the baby's growth with ultrasound in the last ten to twelve weeks of the

pregnancy to make sure that there are no potential problems before birth.

For hypothyroidism:
- Treatment is with supplements of thyroid hormone in the form of thyroxine tablets taken daily. They are safe to take in pregnancy and during breastfeeding – the thyroid hormone occurs naturally in your body, after all.
- Your thyroid hormone levels are usually tested during pregnancy and the dosage of thyroxine adjusted if necessary. Should dosage adjustment be required during your pregnancy, review it after delivery in case your hormone levels have changed.

did you know?

Some risk factors for venous thrombosis in pregnancy include:
- being over the age of 35
- being overweight
- immobility (which leads to sluggish blood flow)
- delivery by Caesarean section
- severe varicose veins
- pre-eclampsia
- previous DVT
- an inborn tendency for the blood to clot (thrombophilia)
- paraplegia
- sickle-cell disease
- infection
- dehydration
- long-distance travel

Venous thrombosis

A venous thrombosis is simply a blood clot in the vein, the vast majority of which occur in the leg veins. In pregnant women, most clots arise in the left leg, usually at the top of the leg or in the pelvis, whereas in non-pregnant women, they most often arise in the veins in the calf muscles of either leg. The most serious type of clot is the deep venous thrombosis (DVT), which lies deep within the leg muscles. A DVT is troublesome, particularly when some of the clot breaks off and travels to the lung where it can block part of the circulation. This is known as a pulmonary thromboembolism and can be life-threatening. Although death in such cases is rare, it is the most frequent cause of mothers dying in pregnancy in the UK. It is therefore important to try to prevent DVT before it occurs or to treat it before it becomes life threatening.

If you have had a previous DVT, your risk of another is increased during pregnancy, especially if no cause was found, if you have had more than one clot or if you have a thrombophilia, an inborn tendency to clot that can run in families (see box, right). Many doctors believe that women with a previous clot should be tested for thrombophilia prior to conception. This requires a simple blood test and ideally should be done before you get pregnant. Consult your doctor for pre-pregnancy advice as treatment might be needed in pregnancy to reduce the risk.

What happens in pregnancy

Clots are caused by a combination of sluggish blood flow, increased clotting tendency of the blood and damage to the veins, although all three of these factors do not need to be present for a clot to occur. In pregnancy, there is a marked reduction in the speed of the blood flow through the leg veins. This reduced rate of blood flow is present from 16 weeks and is maximal at term. It takes around six weeks to return to normal after you have the baby.

The blood-clotting system also changes in pregnancy, with increased levels of clotting factors in the blood – it is believed that this is how your body prepares for any blood loss at delivery. However, this also leads to an increased tendency of the blood to clot when you are pregnant. Minor damage to the veins in the pelvis can easily occur at the time of delivery as the baby presses on these veins. Because of these changes, the risk of having a clot increases when you are pregnant and

watch out!
The body has natural systems to stop excessive clotting. Some people are born with a tendency for these systems not to work properly, which gives them an increased risk of blood clots. This condition is called thrombophilia and it comes in many forms. Often there is a family history of thrombosis because thrombophilia can be a genetic problem that is passed down through the generations.

particularly after delivery. However, only about 1:1,000 women get a venous thrombosis during their pregnancy.

Leg pain and marked swelling, especially in a woman with risk factors for thrombosis, is the usual way that a blood clot first comes to light. However, many pregnant women already have swollen legs in pregnancy and some discomfort is not uncommon also. So leg swelling in pregnancy is not usually caused by a DVT. If the doctor is concerned that you might have a clot in your leg, a specific test (usually an ultrasound scan), is carried out to determine if there is a blood clot in the large vein at the top of the leg.

Treatment in pregnancy

If you have had only one previous DVT with no underlying thrombophilia, then it is essential to weigh up all the risk factors for your particular case to determine if you need heparin treatment. This is a highly specialized area and specific advice about your particular situation must be obtained from a specialist.

Treatment in pregnancy is similar to what you would receive when you are not pregnant: a medication called heparin, which is an anticoagulant that 'thins' the blood. It offers no risk to the developing baby. Heparin is not effective if given by mouth so it has to be injected and most women can be taught to inject themselves without any difficulty.

In non-pregnant women with a thrombosis, heparin treatment is followed by warfarin, another anticoagulant. However, warfarin freely crosses the placenta and can cause problems in the baby. Wherever possible, doctors will avoid prescribing warfarin in pregnancy. It is safe to switch to warfarin following delivery as almost none of this medication gets into breast milk.

Although heparin offers no risk to the developing baby, there have been some potential side effects on the mother during pregnancy.

• With use over several months there is a small risk of heparin-induced osteoporosis or thinning of the bones.

• Occasionally an allergic reaction to heparin can also occur. In recent years, a newer form of heparin – known as low-molecular-weight heparin – has been used, which has fewer side effects and a much lower risk of osteoporosis.

Want to know more?

Websites for additional info

ACeBabes support on pregnancy following fertility treatment
www.acebabes.co.uk

Action on pre-eclampsia http://www.apec.org.uk/

British Infertility Counselling Association (BICA) www.bica.net

British Medical Association
http://www.bma.org.uk/ap.nsf/Content/AZusefulsites

Childlessness Overcome Through Surrogacy (COTS) www.surrogacy.org.uk

Donor Conception Network www.dcnetwork.org

Ectopic Pregnancy Trust http://www.ectopic.org

Family Planning Association http://www.fpa.org.uk/

Fertility Friends http://www.fertilityfriends.co.uk/

HFEA http://www.hfea.gov.uk/cps/rde/xchg/hfea

Infertility Network UK www.infertilitynetworkuk.com

Miscarriage Association www.miscarriageassociation.org.uk

Multiple Births Foundation www.multiplebirths.org.uk

National Childbirth Trust (NCT) www.nctpregnancyandbabycare.com

National Electronic Library for Health (NHS) http://www.library.nhs.uk

National Endometriosis Society www.endo.org.uk

National Gamete Donation Trust www.ngdt.co.uk

National Institute for Clinical Excellence (NICE) www.nice.org.uk

Pink Parents UK www.pinkparents.org.uk

Stillbirth and Neonatal Death Society (SANDS) www.uk-sands.org

Royal College of Obstetricians and Gynecologists http://www.rcog.org.uk

Scottish Care and Information on Miscarriage
http://www.miscarriagesupport.org.uk/

Surrogacy UK www.surrogacyuk.org

Twins and Multiple Births Association (TAMBA) www.tamba.org.uk

Verity (for women with polycystic ovarian syndrome) www.verity-pcos.org.uk

Index